MEDICINA CLASSICA

GUY PATIN

(*Frontispiece*)

GUY PATIN FROM "LETTRES CHOISIES." PARIS: JEAN PETIT. 1685.

GUY PATIN

AND THE MEDICAL PROFESSION IN PARIS IN THE XVIIth CENTURY

By

FRANCIS R. PACKARD, M.D.
Author of Life and Times of Ambroise Pare
Editor of Annals of Medical History

WITH SEVENTEEN ILLUSTRATIONS
INCLUDING NINE FULL PAGE PLATES

AUGUSTUS M. KELLEY · PUBLISHERS
NEW YORK 1970

First Published 1924
(New York: Paul B. Hoeber, Inc.)

Reprinted 1970 By
AUGUSTUS M. KELLEY, PUBLISHERS
NEW YORK, NEW YORK 10001

SBN 678 03759 0

Library of Congress Catalogue Card Number
78-95624

Printed in the United States of America

INTRODUCTION

THE formerly so-celebrated correspondence of Guy Patin, and even his name have fallen recently into such undeserved oblivion that it seems timely to the writer that an attempt should be made to revive interest in this famous old French worthy, whose letters written during a period of over forty years (1630–1672) give us such an invaluable picture of the life of the times, not only from the medical point of view but in all its aspects, military, religious, political and courtly. As the great French critic, Sainte-Beuve, wrote of Patin's letters:

> One finds in these letters, *bon mots*, the news of the day, many curious details on the literature and learned men of the time, above all a lucid and natural manner, with free, bold traits, which point to the life, the mind, the genius of the author. It is a conversation without design, without pretention, often sportive. They are the confidences of one friend to another, full of crudity, of passion, sometimes of grossness, often of good sense, humor, and salt of every kind.

Bayle, in his "Dictionnaire biographique," warns that "it is necessary to read his letters with distrust because most of the political and literary anecdotes in them are false or ill-founded," and Voltaire says of them:

His collection of letters has been read with avidity because it contained new anecdotes which everybody loves, and satires which one loves even more. It serves to show how much contemporary authors who write precipitately the news of the day are unfaithful guides for history. Such news is often false or disfigured by malignity and moreover this multitude of petty details is scarcely of value save to small minds.

These criticisms may be true as to the historic value of Patin's letters, nevertheless, as pictures of the life of the day they are invaluable and it must be remembered Guy did not purpose writing history when he penned them.

Reveillé-Parise quotes a statement made by Fontenelle, the nephew of Corneille and himself a distinguished litterateur, who was born in 1657, and thus grew up among men who had known Patin personally. In his eulogy of Denis Dodart, Fontenelle says: "All the circumstances testified to by

M. Patin are worthy of attention. He was a physician, very learned and passionate for the glory of medicine. He wrote to a friend not only with entire but sometimes with excessive liberty. Eulogies are not very frequent in his letters, that which dominates them being a very independent philosophic bile."

Guy did not write his letters for publication. The first edition was not published, fortunately for him, until he had been in his grave eleven years, and was consequently immune from the vengeance of those whom he so bitterly offended by the freedom of his language. It is to this that, with all due allowance for his individual prejudices, which were violent and doubtless unreasonable, the great value of the correspondence is due. He wrote of persons and events with a liberty, not to say license, which he would certainly not have dared use had he thought his letters would see the light of day, especially as the chief objects of his attacks were those high in place, such as Richelieu and Mazarin, or powerful organizations, such as the Jesuits, or the Apothecaries. He is equally caustic and personal in his remarks about many of the royal family and the nobility, and this at a time when such writings, if discovered, would have brought severe punishment on their author. Of his own works which were intended for publication Patin says:[1]

> Posterity will forego my writings, likewise I have not much desire to leave any of them. There are two sorts of men who write, the wise and the fools, and I know myself to be neither the one nor the other. Furthermore the life that we lead at Paris is too agitated. The practice of our profession takes from us that tranquillity which it is necessary to have when one wishes to write for eternity.

Elsewhere[2] he urges Spon to make "*un beau* sacrifice to Vulcan, to burn his letters."

Patin's correspondents were chiefly physicians who were like him interested in literary matters.

The earliest letters we have were addressed to the Belins, father and son, each named Claude, who practiced medicine at Troyes. The two Spons were physicians at Lyons. They likewise were father and son. Charles Spon, the elder, was born at Lyons on December 25, 1609, and practiced medicine there until his death on February

[1] Letter to Spon, November 8, 1658.
[2] Letter of January 8, 1650.

21, 1684. In spite of his very large practice he was the author of a number of books. Reveillé-Parise says his most important work was an edition of the "Aphorisms and Prognostics of Hippocrates" which he dedicated to Patin.

Jacques Spon, the son of Charles, was born at Lyons in 1647. Although a physician he seems to have been interested chiefly in antiquarian research. In company with an Englishman named Vehler, he traveled extensively through southeastern Europe, Greece and Turkey, and published a "Relation" of his travels. As he was a Huguenot he retired into Switzerland where he died in extreme poverty in 1685, the year of the Revocation of the Edict of Nantes.

André Falconet, Patin's correspondent, was of a distinguished line of physicians. His father, Charles Falconet, was physician to Marguerite of Valois, the first wife of Henri IV. André was born at Lyons, November 12, 1612 and died in 1691. He practiced medicine at Lyons with great success. The Letters contain many references to his son, Noël Falconet,[3] who was sent to Paris to study medicine, and lived there with

[3] November 16, 1644–May 14, 1724.

Patin as his house pupil. Noël had a son, Camille Falconet, who after practicing at Lyons moved to Paris where he attained great distinction, not only as a physician, but as a booklover. His history sounds very much as if some of the spirit of his father's preceptor had been transmitted to him. Camille died at Paris in 1762.

The formal writings of Guy Patin were not numerous and it must be confessed that their interest was mostly ephemeral. They will be found listed in an appended bibliography, and if one will take the trouble to read such of them as are available, he will arise from their perusal with the conviction that Patin's fame must rest on his correspondence and not on such evidences of his erudition or medical skill as are contained in his professional writings.

This is not the sole instance in which an individual's posthumous fame has arisen from some other attribute than that to which he personally would have wished the greater importance attached.

As occurs with all unauthorized or surreptitious publications the correspondence has undergone many vicissitudes in the various editions in which it has been preserved to us. Triaire,[4] in the preface to the edition which he undertook to publish in 1907 and which he intended to be complete and definitive, summarily reviews the many defects which appertain to each of them. He says:

The editors have not contented themselves with throwing aside at their convenience a considerable quantity of unpublished documents, but they have also not hesitated to suppress numerous passages in those which they have published. They have gone further yet and have not recoiled before alterations of the text, before falsification of the ideas of the author. They have altered his manuscript, replacing a strong and exact expression, such as he threw it from his pen, by a dull or insignificant word; modifying at their will entire passages, giving résumés of these passages instead of their complete text: attaching, after cutting out without limit, two or three letters together, or on the other hand dividing one letter into many and forging from the pieces patchworks more or less ingenious to supply the solutions of continuity which result from such actions. All the editions, of which the greater part are based on one another, reproduce the errors of

[4] Lettres de Gui Patin, 1630–1672. Nouvelle édition collectionée sur les manuscrits autographes, etc. Paris, 1907.

their predecessors in adding to them faults of their own, not excepting the last, the only modern one, that of 1846, due to M. Reveillé-Parise.

After this severe arraignment M. Triaire relates the several efforts that have been made to collate the letters with the object of publishing a definitive edition. In 1760 M. Formy, perpetual secretary of the Academy of Berlin, conceived the project but for some reason not stated his plan aborted. In 1846 Reveillé-Parise published an edition at Paris in three volumes for which he claimed completeness and accuracy, but which Triaire following Sainte-Beuve condemns for inaccuracy and incompleteness.

In 1895 MM. de Montaiglon and Tamisey de la Roque had gathered together all the available letters with a mass of correlative information, notes, etc., when the entire collection was destroyed by fire.

Finally Triaire himself, undaunted by the failures of his predecessors, undertook the task and gave to the world in 1907 one volume of what he promised to make the long sought for definitive edition.

Unfortunately Triaire has only published one volume of his edition, and in the correspondence therein contained there are only the letters written up to March, 1649. He has arranged these letters consecutively, according to date, whereas Reveillé-Parise has collected the letters into groups according to the person to whom they were written. Triaire's arrangement is preferable.

In 1911 Pierre Pic published a most delightful collection of selections from the correspondence[5] with a learned and interesting introduction, in which while admitting the great value of the "letters" from the historic and literary point of view he deprecates the style in which they are written and says that when Sainte-Beuve wrote his praise of them he seems not to have been struck by the "two principal defects of Patin, the eternal idle talk, and the ferocious scolding for all that which is not his personal opinion." Pic criticizes Patin's habit of interlarding his letters with Latin, which he says he does not do judiciously and correctly after the manner of Montaigne, but in a foolishly pedantic and often inaccurate way. For those who wish to read what is best of Patin and to acquire the real flavor of his "letters"

[5] Guy Patin avec 74 portraits ou documents. Paris, G. Steinheil, 1911.

there is no better edition of them than Pic's, which will certainly stimulate the reader to further researches on their author.

Triaire[6] states:

The original letters of Patin to the Belins of Troyes are contained in the manuscript inscribed at the Bibliothèque Nationale under the number 9,538 (Fonds Français. Suppl. Français, 2,034, *bis*). This manuscript contains 175 letters addressed to Belin *père et fils*—of which one is not in the hand of the author but bears his signature; twenty-eight letters to Spon, of which five have been likewise written by another pen but are signed by Patin; a letter without any address, but manifestly destined to Spon; and one addressed to Charpentier, physician of the Faculty of Paris. An inscription indicates that the manuscript came from the sale of M. Gay of Lyons, in 1634. Pic[7] states that there is in the Library of the Faculté de Médecine in Paris a collection of 459 letters written by Patin to a number of foreign scientists, among whom he mentions Thomas Bartholin of Copenhagen, Meibomius and Van der Linden of Leyden, Scheffer of Frankfort, Gaspard Bauhin of Bâle, and Volckamer of Nuremberg. The letters are written in Latin

[6] Lettres de Gui Patin, Libraire Honoré Champion. Paris, 1907.

[7] Pic, P. Guy Patin, Paris, 1911.

and the earliest bears the date March 26, 1652, and the latest April 4, 1669. The letters in this collection are not the originals, but copies, some of them by Patin himself, others by his eldest son, Robert, who acted as his secretary. These letters are unpublished.

Triaire states that there is a manuscript in the Library of Wiesbaden entitled "Borbonia ou singularités remarquables prises des conversations des Messieurs Nic. Bourbon et Guy Patin." It is accompanied by the following recommendations addressed by Patin to his son, Charles:

My son, I talk to you as though this was my testament. All these papers which you see here are a farrago, a potpourri thrown in a heap without order, of a quantity of very various things that I have learned or heard spoken of by one person or another; but the greater part comes from a talk which I have continued for many years *cum Viro Clarissimo et Doctissimo Nicolao Borbonio* in the Oratory at Paris. There are some points very free and delicate as much of religion as of the government of princes. All that which I have said of the Jesuits, believe as very true but do not repeat unless it be à propos. . . . I again repeat and recommend to you, read (these papers) and burn them sooner than lend them to anyone.

Nicolas Bourbon, a canon of the Oratory in Paris, was a very learned man and a great friend of Patin's. He was the center of a learned circle which used to meet at the Oratory. Part of the above mentioned manuscript was published with the title "Borboniana."

A curious fact is that Pic transcribes a similar recommendation addressed by Patin to his son which he says precedes the unpublished letters in the Bibliothèque de la Faculté de Médecine. The latter collection was deposited at the École de Santé at Paris by Peyrihle in 1794. Triaire says that M. Ricci stated that the Wiesbaden collection was there in 1907.

Is the Wiesbaden collection the original, of which the letters at Paris are the contemporary copies by Patin and his son?

FRANCIS R. PACKARD.

PHILADELPHIA, PA.

TABLE OF CONTENTS

LIST OF ILLUSTRATIONS

GUY PATIN

AND THE MEDICAL PROFESSION IN PARIS IN THE XVIIth CENTURY

CHAPTER I

Historical Foreword

Patin's life covers a most interesting period in the history of France. He was born in 1601, and was a boy of nine when Henri IV was assassinated, and he died in 1672 when Louis XIV was at the height of his glory. In order to appreciate his letters and their bearing on current events we must comprehend somewhat of the great changes which took place in the social and political life of France in that period.

During the latter half of the sixteenth century France was torn asunder by the religious wars between the Catholics and the Huguenots. After Henri III was assassinated at Saint Cloud in 1589, there were five years more of bitter warfare before Henri

IV succeeded in winning Paris "by a mass" and entered that city as King of France. At last civil peace was restored and under the wise and conservative government of the new king and his great minister, Sully, the internal wounds of France healed rapidly with the marvelous recuperative power which she has shown on so many different occasions in her history. A new era dawned. Men were at liberty to worship according to the dictates of their conscience, the Edict of Nantes, promulgated by Henri IV in 1598, having granted the Huguenots freedom of worship. With peace came prosperity, growth of commerce and agriculture, with corresponding social and intellectual development. The murder of Henri IV, by the dagger of the fanatic, Ravaillac, on May 14, 1610, temporarily interrupted this happy state of affairs.

Henri IV was succeeded by his son, Louis XIII, a boy of nine years. Until he should reach his majority the affairs of the kingdom were placed in the hands of the Queen Mother, Marie de' Medici, who was completely controlled by an Italian named Concini and his wife, Leonora Galigai, who had been Marie de' Medici's foster-sister. Possessed with rapacity and abmition they not only accumulated vast sums of money from the treasury, but Concini had himself made Marquis of Ancre, and although he had never been on a battlefield, Marshal of France. Sully was ignominiously dismissed from the council and the regulation of the affairs of the kingdom lay entirely in the hands of these unscrupulous Italians. Henri IV had accumulated in the royal treasury vast sums which the Queen Regent squandered in gifts on her favorites and in pensions on the leaders of the French nobility whom she endeavored to reconcile in this manner to the domination of Concini. Although she gave with a lavish hand it did not suffice to repress their discontent or political ambitions, and revolts broke out on several occasions which were with difficulty suppressed by the Queen Regent's bestowing enormous sums of money on the leaders, such as Condé, Mayenne, and de Rohan. In 1615, the young King married Anne of Austria. Finally in 1617, when Louis was sixteen years old, resenting the manner in which his mother and Concini excluded him from affairs and inspired by deep personal hatred of the latter, he entered into a conspiracy with his favorite de Luynes, a young man of small ability and little conscience, and Vitry, the Captain of his Guards. Concini was seized by Vitry as he was entering the Louvre and, as he resisted arrest, was instantly killed. His wife was arrested and accused of acquiring influence over the Queen by practicing sorcery. She was found guilty, beheaded and her body burned. Louis declared the regency at an end and placed de Luynes at the head of affairs, but the pride of the old French nobility rebelled against the overwhelming insolence and rapacity of this parvenu as much as it did against that of his predecessor, and they took arms to overthrow him. De Luynes died of a fever in 1621. After his death the Queen Mother, who had been exiled from the court to Blois, became reconciled with the King and with her return to court, Richelieu, whom she had first introduced into public affairs, came into power, and until his death in 1642 was the predominant influence in the affairs of France. To Patin he was the personification of all that was evil, and Patin was only one of many who hated the Cardinal and sought in many ways to accomplish his overthrow. Patin's hatred was partly personal, and as his passions or prejudices were violent in all things so his detestation of Richelieu's government may be

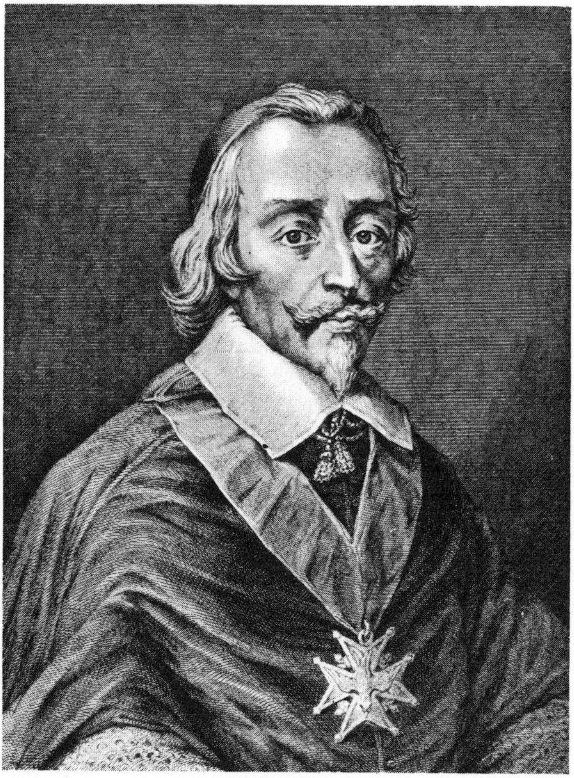

Cardinal de Richelieu
(1585–1642)

largely traced to the fact that at the time of the conspiracy of Cinq-Mars in 1642, Richelieu had executed as one of the conspirators, de Thou, the son of the historian, a great friend of Patin's. However that may be, Patin lets no opportunity slip for delivering himself of the bitterest diatribes against the Cardinal. It is very difficult to judge Richelieu with impartiality. Coming into power at a time when France was fast slipping into the old evil of civil war, the great nobles all heading armed factions, he managed to weather the storms and finally place the real power where it belonged in the hands of the King. The Huguenots and Catholics maintained a condition of armed neutrality, and minor conflicts occurred from time to time which kept up the smouldering enmity. The internal dissensions of France had weakened her standing with other nations, and her military strength was at the lowest ebb. In the few years since the death of Henri IV, agriculture and commerce had been again disturbed by civil commotions and the improvements and reforms instituted by Sully and his great master were neglected.

One of his first measures was to abase the growing power of the Huguenots.

By the Edict of Nantes the Huguenots had been granted certain cities, among them La Rochelle. The latter they had converted into a powerful fortress, supported by a large fleet and army. Richelieu determined to suppress this focus of Protestantism. Taking advantage of an uprising of the Huguenots, Richelieu laid siege to La Rochelle, and after a siege of fifteen months he entered the town in triumph, thereby breaking the military power of the Huguenots in France forevermore. Their military power broken Richelieu treated the Protestants with an astonishing liberality, permitting them to hold their religious beliefs and services, to practice the liberal professions, and even to hold high offices in the army and navy and in political and civil life. Richelieu determined from an early day to check the power of the nobility. In 1626 the comte de Chalais having entered into a conspiracy with a number of others to dethrone Louis XIII and make his brother, Gaston d'Orléans, king, Richelieu arrested a number of the greatest persons at the Court. The comte de Chalais was beheaded, the duchesse de Chevreuse, the most intimate friend of the Queen, was exiled, some natural sons of Henri IV who had entered into the conspiracy were imprisoned in the Bastille, and the duc d'Orléans forced to make the most abject professions of loyalty. The most stringent edicts had been promulgated against duelling. They were set at defiance by the nobility until in 1627 when Richelieu had two nobles, the comte de Bouteville and the comte de Chapelle, executed at the Place de la Grève for fighting a duel. Even the Queen Mother, to whom Richelieu owed his start in power, had to succumb to the terrible Cardinal. In 1630 she persuaded Louis, by working on his fears and jealousy, to disgrace the Cardinal. The latter left the Court and the courtiers all hastened to the apartments of the Queen Mother to congratulate her and to ingratiate themselves. But the King repented in a few hours and Richelieu was recalled. The day was known subsequently as the Day of Dupes, but those who had deceived themselves were bitterly awakened to their error. The Queen Mother was sent away from the Court to Compiègne, whence she fled to Brussels, dying an exile in 1631. The *garde des sceaux*, Marillac, and his brother, who was a Marshal of France, were arrested. The *garde des sceaux* died in prison and the Marshal was beheaded. Bassompierre, the future Marshal of France, was put in the Bastille for twelve years. Gaston d'Orléans went to Brussels to join the Queen Mother. There they concocted a new rebellion in conjunction with the duc de Montmorency. The royal forces defeated the army of the rebels at Castelnaudary in 1632. Gaston ran away, and the duc de Montmorency was executed.

In 1642 the comte de Cinq-Mars attempted a conspiracy to overthrow Richelieu. It has been suspected, though never proved, that the King was party to the plot. It was discovered and Cinq Mars, with the other leaders, was executed. Thus Richelieu destroyed the last vestige of feudalism. The Fronde was only a phantom of the former uprisings of the nobility.

On December 1, 1642, to the savagely expressed joy of Patin, the Cardinal died.

Richelieu was fond of literature. He founded the Académie Française in 1635, and rebuilt the Sorbonne. He also established the royal printing press and the Jardin des Plantes, the latter being especially designed as an aid to medical science. Richelieu built and lived in the Palais Royal, then known as the Palais Cardinal.

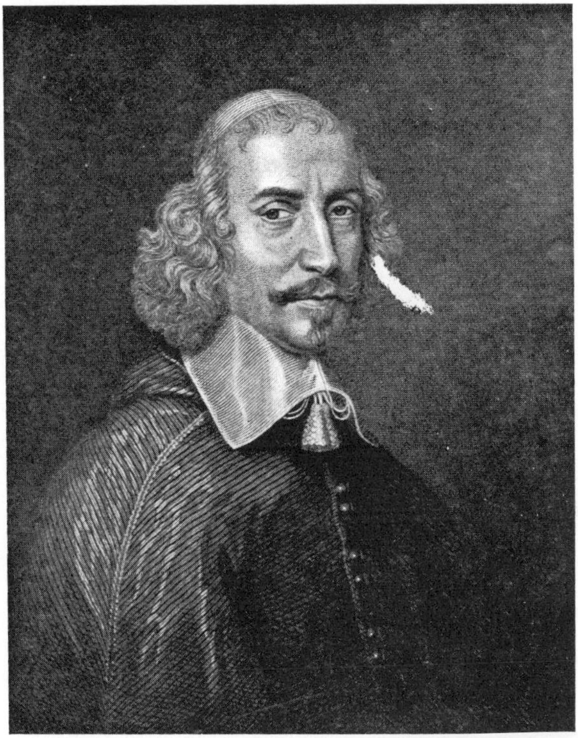

Cardinal Mazarin
(1602–1661)

Louis XIII only survived his great minister about six months, dying on May 14, 1643. Once more the throne of France was left to an infant, Louis XIV, aged less than five years, with the regency in the hands of a Queen Mother, Anne of Austria, and strange to say with another cardinal, Mazarin, an Italian by birth, as chief minister. Mazarin had been brought forward by Richelieu and proved a worthy pupil although undoubtedly not as able or great a man as his predecessor. There is much ground for the belief that Mazarin was secretly married to Anne of Austria or at any rate that he was her lover.

The early years of the new reign were marked by the victories of the great Condé and Turenne, over the Spaniards and Germans in the course of the Thirty Years' War, which dragged on its weary way from 1618 until the Peace of Westphalia in 1648, by which France secured possession of Alsace. The finances of the country were in a terrible condition at this time. The superintendent of finances, Particelli d'Esmery, was a corrupt Italian. His extravagance and venality necessitated the most onerous taxation. Mazarin was much more avaricious than Richelieu, amassing enormous wealth for himself and his relatives. Places at the court and government positions, as well as in the army and navy, were openly sold, and we can read in Patin's letters the way in which positions in the medical service of the court were sold to the highest bidder, regardless of merit. Mazarin either got all, or a large part of most of the bargains thus made. The Parlement of Paris had become a center of opposition to the corruption and venality of the court. Mazarin resolved in August, 1648, to break the opposition by seizing three of the members who had taken the most active part. They were named de Blancmesnil, Broussel, and Charton. The last named ran away, de Blancmesnil was easily taken prisoner, but when some guards had put Broussel in a coach to carry him off, a clamor was raised and the population of Paris rose in revolt. The Parlement of Paris marched to the Louvre followed by an immense mob. After a brief show of resistance the Court yielded and the arrested magistrates were released.

This insurrection and that of the Fronde which developed immediately afterwards were fomented largely by the activity of Paul de Gondi, later Cardinal de Retz, the coadjutor to the Archbishop of Paris. He was intelligent, wealthy, unscrupulous, and above all a demagogue. Mazarin and the Queen Mother determined at the first auspicious moment to renew the fight, when they felt themselves in a stronger position. Accordingly, in February, 1649, the Queen Mother, with the King and Mazarin, left Paris and went to Saint-Germain, where the prince de Condé, always known as le Grand Condé in French history because of his illustrious military services, took command of the troops which remained loyal, and war was declared on the Parlement of Paris and the rebellious populace. Many of the nobility hastened to Paris to take part with the people, among them the prince de Conti, younger brother of the Great Condé, the duc de Longueville, the duc de Bouillon, and the duc de Beaufort. The latter, a grandson of Henri IV, had received the nickname of the *roi des halles*, or king of the markets, because of his popularity with the market women of Paris and the lowest class of the people. He was very handsome, with affable manners but absolutely devoid of capacity. The prince de Conti was chosen commander of the peoples' army. The coadjutor de

Retz displayed the most feverish activity in stirring up the rebellion and maintaining the spirits of the party. He raised a regiment of cavalry which was dubbed in ridicule the regiment of Corinth because de Retz was titular bishop of Corinth. This civil war on a small scale received the name of the Fronde because of a game which was very popular with the children of that epoch in France. It consisted of throwing stones at one another by means of an instrument like a slingshot, made of a piece of leather between two strings. The police having forbidden this amusement the boys were in the habit of using their weapons on the officers who chased them. Hence those who were opposed to the authorities received the name of Frondeurs.

The so-called war, as Voltaire says, would have been entirely ridiculous had it not been participated in by a king of France, and the Great Condé, and involved the capital of the kingdom. The peoples' troops made many sorties from Paris, which were uniformly repulsed. On their return they would be hooted and jeered at by their fellow-citizens for whose cause they had gone forth to fight. The Parlement having ordered that each house having a porte-cochère should furnish a man and a horse for the service, the cavalry raised by the city in this way was known as the cavalry of the porte-cochères. The popular cause suffered because the nobility who had attached themselves to it were not animated by any real desire to further it, but only by selfish ambition and vanity coupled with personal hatred of the Cardinal and Queen Mother. The contemporary revolution in England succeeded because the men who participated in it were united in an earnest resolve to correct abuses. In France though the abuses existed there was a lack of unity among the groups of the peoples' party which, coupled with the unscrupulous ambition and levity of those who were chosen as its leaders, soon led to its disintegration. Some of the nobility actually attempted to negotiate with Spain, then at war with France, for aid against the Mazarinists, as they preferred to designate their antagonists. It must be remembered that the Parlement of Paris was not at all similar to the institution bearing the name parliament in England. In France the term "parlement" was applied to bodies which existed at Paris, Bordeaux and elsewhere in France, composed of lawyers and prominent bourgeois of the several districts in which they were constituted. They were not only legislative but also judicial bodies. The Parlement of Paris awoke to a realization that their cause was being betrayed by the nobility. Condé had wisely refrained from any serious attack on the city of Paris, contenting himself with merely repulsing the irregular militia which sallied from time to time from its walls. The Parlement entered into negotiations with the King's party and an agreement was soon signed by which the King granted certain concessions, and Paris opened its gates in April, 1649, for the return of the court. As usual the great nobles who had participated on the popular side were easily brought over to the King by the bestowal of money and places. The reconciliation was of short duration. The Great Condé offended Mazarin and the Queen Mother by constantly reminding them that they owed their return to power to him, and he alienated the Parlement and bourgeois by the contempt with which he uniformly treated them. In January, 1650, Mazarin arrested Condé, his brother, the prince de Conti and the duc de Longueville and put them in prison at Vincennes. At first this arrest of the leaders of both factions seemed to please the fickle populace, but the arrogance of Mazarin soon reunited the two factions against him, and instigated by Gondi, to whom Mazarin had promised a cardinal's hat but had not fulfilled his promise, the Fronde rushed into a new revolt. This time they achieved a temporary success, forcing the Queen Mother in February, 1651, to liberate Condé, Conti and de Longueville, and to exile Mazarin from France. Mazarin went to Cologne but from that city continued to influence the Queen Regent. Gondi at last secured the long desired cardinal's hat, but the Great Condé was dissatisfied with the result of the revolt. He was liberated from prison but instead of finding himself at the head of affairs he soon realized that Mazarin yet controlled them from his place of exile, by his power over the Queen Mother. This great soldier then became a traitor. He entered into a treaty with the Spaniards and raised an armed force against the King. Mazarin was hastily summoned back to Paris by Anne of Austria and the famous General Turenne was given command of the royal troops. At first Condé was successful. The Court fled from Paris. Finally both the royal army under Turenne, and the rebel army under Condé approached Paris, each demanding that the city open its gates to them. The Parisians refused entrée to both. Gaston, duc d'Orléans, with his daughter the famous Mademoiselle, and the Cardinal de Retz were in the city. The royal troops and the rebels fought a battle in the Faubourg Saint-Antoine, and Mademoiselle ordered the cannon of the Bastille to fire on the royal troops, and the gates of the city to be opened to Condé's army. The latter entered the city, but finding he could not hold it retired and led his army to join the Spanish troops in Flanders. The party of the King and Mazarin triumphed. The Cardinal was more powerful and arrogant than ever. The duc d'Orléans was exiled to Blois, de Retz was imprisoned, Condé sentenced to death in contumacy, and a royal edict forbade the Parlement henceforth to attempt any interference in affairs of state or finance. The war with Spain was carried on. Mazarin entered into an alliance with Oliver Cromwell, the Protestant ruler who had beheaded the king whose wife was the daughter of Henri IV. Peace was finally made in 1659. As part of its terms Condé was pardoned and Louis XIV married the Infanta Marie Thérèse.

Mazarin was as bitterly hated by Patin as Richelieu had been. He inveighs against his arrogance, his avarice and the way in which he provided for the welfare of his family at the expense of France. Even the splendid library founded by Mazarin for the use of men of letters, of which Patin's friend Gabriel Naudé was librarian, and the establishment of the College of the Four Nations at the University of Paris designed to provide for scholars from Spain, Italy, Germany and the Low Countries, could not make Patin see any good in this *chaperon rouge*. The letters express nothing but hatred and contempt towards him. Mazarin died on March 9, 1661.

The last decade of Patin's life corresponds with the first ten years of the personal reign of Louis XIV. While Mazarin lived he was the dominant power in the kingdom, but after his death Louis could truthfully state: "L'état, c'est moi." One of the earliest manifestations of his desire for absolute control was the disgrace of Fouquet.[1]

[1] Those who are readers of Dumas will recall the Vicomte de Bragelonne, in which romance the disgrace of Fouquet forms the principal theme. The Letters of Madame de Sévigné contain much information about his trial.

Fouquet as minister of finance, though a man of superior ability, had thrown the finances into extreme disorder, by reckless extravagance. He had accumulated an immense personal fortune. In 1661 he gave a magnificent fête to the King at his superb château de Vaux, the glories of which outshone those of the royal palaces. The King was angered at the display, but it was probably only the culmination of his discontent at the minister against whom Colbert had for some time been arousing the King's suspicions. A few weeks later in September, 1661, Fouquet was arrested. His trial continued for three years. At the end he was found guilty. Nine judges wished him executed, thirteen were for imprisonment for life. Fouquet had been a great patron of letters. La Fontaine, Pellisson, Mademoiselle de Scudéry and Madame de Sévigné all owed much to his patronage and have defended his memory. His place was given to Colbert, under whose able administration was finally grouped not only the finances, but also the direction of the beaux-arts, agriculture, commerce, public works and the navy. Patin naturally sympathized with Fouquet. He termed Colbert a "man of marble" and could see no good in one of the greatest of the great ministers of Louis XIV.

Another man who contributed much to the glory of the reign of the *roi soleil* was Louvois, his minister of war. He was the first to ordain a distinctive military uniform for the different units of the army; to introduce the use of the bayonet attached to the musket; to organize magazines for the storage of powder, arms and munitions in different places whence they could be readily distributed in case of need, and he organized the army into special divisions: cavalry, artillery, infantry, and subdivided these again into special bodies trained for their various duties: dragoons, hussards, grenadiers, fusileers, etc. He also established a special corps of engineers and first brought into use portable pontoon bridges, and he was the first to arrange for camps of maneuvre in times of peace. Under Louvois the great military engineer, Vauban, constructed the fortifications along the frontier which for so many generations held the external enemies of France in check. Vauban was the greatest master of fortification and of the construction of siege works and his ideas and inventions completely changed the methods of making war.

To the military successes of Louis XIV, Colbert contributed greatly by his able administration of the navy. Mazarin had left this important arm in a deplorable condition. Colbert built up a wonderful merchant marine and used it as a feeder for the establishment of a navy which soon rendered France a formidable power at sea. He brought foreign shipbuilders to work on the construction of new warships, and built huge yards at various ports. Schools of navigation, of hydrography, and of naval warfare were established. Rank in the navy was established in order to attract men of birth and intelligence, and an *inscription maritime* or naval reserve was organized among the maritime population. In external affairs the glory of France was equally well maintained by an able minister, de Pionne, who died in 1671, the year before Patin's death. Spain was in a decadence which the ambition of Philip II had begun. Italy was constantly at war. Germany was in the same chaotic condition and Austria so weak that she was obliged to appeal for aid to repel the menaces of the Turks. England had just restored the Stuarts. Holland was the richest and actually the most menacing of the rival countries, chiefly because of its naval power. Louis XIV availed himself skilfully of the weaknesses of her neighbors to aggrandize France. Though Patin speaks contemptuously of many of the acts by which Louis supported his policy and achieved his objects their success was obvious, and until 1685, the year of the Revocation of the Edict of Nantes, the prosperity of France and the glory of its King steadily increased.

In 1665 Philip IV of Spain died, leaving a son, Charles II, the issue of a second marriage. When Louis XIV was married to Marie Thérèse, Philip's daughter by his first wife, in 1659, it had been stipulated that she should renounce her rights of succession to the Spanish crown and in lieu thereof the Spanish government was to give her a dot of 5,000,000 gold *écus*. Mazarin calculated that Spain would be unable or unwilling to pay this immense sum and that the way would thus be paved for the French to claim the succession. When Philip died in 1665, the dot not having been paid, Louis XIV at once claimed for his wife her rights of succession in the Low Countries, also asserting that as his wife was a minor at the time of her marriage her father had no right to renounce her succession in her name. Upon the refusal of the Spanish government to comply with his demand Louis invaded Flanders in 1667. Its conquest was easy. Town after town yielded. Holland alarmed at this success formed an alliance with England and Sweden, and Louis decided not to proceed further in his triumphal career. The treaty of Aix-la-Chapelle was concluded with Spain in 1668. Louis was bitterly offended by the action of Holland and determined to be avenged on the bourgeois commonwealth. By a large bribe he seduced the Swedes from the alliance. His brother, Philippe d'Orléans, a very worthless individual, had married Henrietta, the sister of Charles II, who was known by the official title of Madame. She was chosen to negotiate with Charles II in 1670 and soon succeeded in persuading and bribing her brother to abandon the Hollanders and enter into an alliance with the French King. On her return to the French court Madame died suddenly. Suspicions of poisoning were at once aroused but they were certainly groundless. Bossuet preached a famous sermon in her honor. The neutrality or aid of the Emperor and the various petty potentates of Germany was secured, and the way being thus prepared, in the spring of 1672 France declared war on Holland. Although the French won great military successes at its outset, this war was the beginning of the misfortunes which darkened the last years of the reign of Louis XIV. Within a few years England and most of his other allies had abandoned him. New alliances were formed to combat his overweening ambition. Against Prince Eugène and Marlborough the French armies sustained a series of terrible defeats. The Prince of Orange, his most determined foe, became King of England and the old French King saw the splendor of his reign sink in an obscuring twilight. By the Revocation of the Edict of Nantes in 1685 France lost 500,000 of her best citizens, and much of her commercial prosperity. Patin died in the spring of 1672 just at the dawning of evil times. During his life he had witnessed the gradual emergence of France from the chaos of the Fronde to the firm although despotic government of an absolute monarch. His letters give many illuminating reflections of the stirring events of which he lived in the very center and many of the chief actors whom he knew. It would have been hard for him to write without bias, and though the pictures he paints are somewhat lurid, they are certainly honest representations of events as he saw them from day to day. Patin was an ardent student of philosophy and theology and his letters are full of information about the Jansenist controversy and the many other disputes with which the learned of the seventeenth century filled so many volumes now condemned to oblivion. It would seem that in his later days the bitterness of political squabbles had been replaced by the *odium theologicum.* Although he was a vigorous opponent of the dominant party, hating the Jesuits and denouncing monks on every possible occasion, he nevertheless managed not to make himself conspicuous enough to undergo any persecution for his opinions, and he apparently died in the Roman Catholic faith and was certainly buried according to its rites.

CHAPTER II

Patin's Youth and Education at the University of Paris

FAMILY AND EDUCATION

As he signed himself frequently "Bellovacensis" (of Beauvais) many writers assert that Patin was a native of that city. Reveillé-Parise says he was born at La Place, a small hamlet in the commune of Hodenc-en-Bray in which the Patin family held a fief from time immemorial, and in 1898 the municipality of La Place erected a monument to his memory. In a letter to Spon (June 14, 1644) Patin himself says that his natal place was a village three leagues from Beauvais in Picardy, named "Houdan" which was the name borne by Hodenc-en-Bray until 1770, and according to Triaire, Guy Patin was born there at the Ferme des Préaux on Friday, August 31, 1601.

His family was typical of the best class of bourgeois. Patin states that he had traced it back for 300 years, during which period some had been notaries at Beauvais, some linen merchants at Paris, some soldiers and others farmers. Patin's grandfather was a soldier "comme tout ce temps-la fut de guerre." His father François had studied law at Orléans and Bourges and would have practiced his profession at Paris had it not been for the death of Henri III, and the siege of Paris which followed thereon. He must have been a Huguenot sympathizer because he had been made a prisoner by the Leaguers and had had to pay a large ransom to secure his release. Guy says that his grandmother had to pledge her wedding jewelry and a belt of silver with a goldsmith at Beauvais to raise the money and that many times he had heard her tell about it, "weeping and detesting the misfortunes of those times."

Patin inherited his parent's hatred for the Guises. The League had been formed by their adherents and they aimed at procuring for their family the succession to the throne, either by the deposition of Henri III or, if not, by successful rebellion in the event of his death, as he had no direct heirs and Henri de Navarre, the nearest in the succession was a Huguenot. Henri III forestalled the plans of the Guises and their League by the murder of the duc Henri de Guise and his brother, the Cardinal. The duc de Guise was known by the nickname Balafré, the scarred, because of a huge cicatrix which disfigured his face. Patin writes Spon (December 24, 1658):

M. de Guise-le-Balafré said formerly:

By war we gain
Credit and money

He was the duc de Guise, who was chief of the League and whom Henri III, by a wise and generous council, caused to be killed at Blois, in the year 1588 on Christmas Eve. My late father, who hated the League and the Leaguers, said when I was yet young, that this massacre was the best coup that this king made in his life.

Gaspard D'Auxy, Seigneur de Monçeaux and Baron de Houdan, recognizing the honesty and ability of François Patin persuaded him to give up his career at the Paris bar and come back to Picardy to manage the business affairs of his family and estate. He made Patin many generous promises which Guy says he did not fulfill. The great man did procure for his man of affairs a virtuous and well-to-do wife of good family, Claude Manessier, having in mind thereby to fix him in the neighborhood and keep him away from Paris; otherwise Guy says that he was ungrateful and avaricious and ruined what would otherwise have been the very successful career of the elder Patin at Paris.

Patin in a letter to Falconet (July 15, 1661) gives another version of the reason his father left Paris. He writes: "My father and mother were good people, who retired to the country to get away from the evil (malice) of Paris, where they lived *ex avito fundulo* until they died."

The Patins had seven children, five daughters and two sons. Guy's brother settled himself in Holland, and the five daughters all married and established themselves with the inheritance of their mother's money. The regret of the father at his own mistaken step, led him to the determination that Guy should fare better.

For this reason he began his son's education at a very early age, one of the steps he took being to cause his son to read Plutarch's "Lives" aloud while he would correct his pronunciation. At the age of nine years he placed him in the Collège at Beauvais, and afterwards sent him to the Collège de Boncourt in Paris, where the boy was for two years a pensionnaire, taking the course in philosophy. An offer of a benefice was made to Patin by some of the nobility. To accept this it was necessary for him to become a priest which he refused to do, thereby greatly angering his mother who did not overcome her resentment for five years, although his father approved his course. A friend of his advised him to study medicine and he did so at Paris from 1622 to 1627 when he received his degree, at which, as he tells us, his mother, as well as his father, was well pleased and helped in the purchase of books and other necessary expenses. Bayle states on the authority of Drélincourt that Patin eked out a living in Paris while pursuing his studies by proof-reading. There is a tradition that the anonymous friend who, Patin says, urged him to study medicine was Riolan, the anatomist of Paris. Riolan is chiefly remembered for the bitterness with which he fought Harvey's demonstration of the circulation. Patin does not refer to him in any way in his autobiographical letter to Spon, in which, from its character, one would think he would have mentioned so great an influence in his life.

This statement is also made in "Naudeana et Patiniana":

By a fatality too common to men of letters he was compelled to become a proof-reader after having received his degree. On seeing some of his corrections, M. Riolan, the celebrated physician, who was regarded among his confrères as the arbiter of reputations, bestowed on him his esteem and friendship, and introduced him to the world.

MEDICAL EDUCATION IN PARIS

The "Letters," as would be expected, are full of references to medical education as it prevailed in the University of Paris. As Minivielle[1] emphasizes, the teaching consisted entirely in the exposition of the works of Hippocrates, Galen and the lesser ancients. There was no attempt at clinical instruction; and medical learning, as manifested by the professors, consisted solely in a display of great erudition in the texts of Greek and Latin authors. In order to enter on the study of medicine in the Faculté de Médecine at the Université de Paris, it was necessary first to possess the degree of Master of Arts or else to have studied philosophy for at least two years, and then there were three steps to the degree, that of bachelor, licentiate and

[1] La médecine au temps d'Henri IV.

finally doctor. After two years study in medicine, if the scholar was twenty-two years old, he could take his examination for his bachelorship. He had to produce first a certificate of good conduct from three physicians, to declare that he belonged to the Catholic Church, and to swear on the Bible that he would be present at the masses said before the Faculté de Médecine. After these formalities were complied with he was questioned during three days on the studies he had pursued and then had to comment on an aphorism of Hippocrates. If he succeeded in passing this ordeal he took an oath that he would defend the decrees, practices, customs and statutes of the Faculty; that he would show respect and honor to the Dean and all the Masters of the Faculty; that he would defend the Faculty against whosoever would undertake anything against its statutes or honor, and above all against those who practiced medicine illegally; and that he would be present in his robes at all the masses ordered by the Faculty, arriving before the end of the Epistle and remaining until the end of the service, and that he would attend the masses for the dead, and the funerals of the Masters (professors) under penalty of a gold crown for failure to do so. Minivielle, whose delightful little book contains the most explicit account of the life of the medical student at Paris in the sixteenth century, states that after having thus been admitted a bachelor in medicine, the student passed the next two years in sustaining theses, studying, sometimes visiting sick persons with the masters, with an occasional opportunity to witness an anatomical demonstration on the human body.

Such opportunities to witness, not actually perform, dissections on the human body must have been very rare, for Patin writes to Charles Spon (May 7, 1657) about a young man who had proposed to visit Paris to study medicine: "If he had come last winter he would have been able to see dissections very easily, because we have never had so many. Four public dissections were held in our schools, of which two were held on women, and more than six by the surgeons, which he could have witnessed."

Saumaise gave an introductory letter to Patin to a young man who wished to study medicine at Paris and Patin writes Spon (December 8, 1649) with what pleasure he would do all he could for the young man because of his admiration for Saumaise:

This is why I have offered him what a certain man promised and offered in Terence, *rem, opem, operam et consilium,* and also money when he wished it. He asks to see anatomical dissections, surgical operations, the debates in our hospitals. He will have all this and more. I have promised to boot to take him to see some patients with me, and that he may attend some of our consultations where among others he will encounter Messieurs Riolan and Moreau.

The bachelors in medicine had to sustain certain theses in public, or as we would now term it, undergo public examinations on medical subjects. These were of two kinds, first the *thèse quodlibétaire*, which might be chosen from any subject in medicine or physiology, on which the candidate was questioned from six in the morning until noon, by nine doctors. The examination was conducted entirely in Latin. Second the *thèse cardinale*, so called after the Cardinal d'Estouteville, who instituted it in 1452, at the time when he was engaged in reforming the teaching at the University of Paris. The *thèse cardinale* was sustained by the candidate for license in much the same manner as the other, but its subject had to appertain to hygiene. Minivielle quotes some of the bizarre and absurd topics utilized as subjects for the theses, such as: "Was the cure of Tobias by the gall of the fish natural?" "Is it salutary to inebriate oneself once a month?" "Are beautiful women more apt to bear children?" "What think you of the saying *in vino veritas?*"

The young man who presented a thesis had not only to sustain his argument but the ideas which he expressed had to be in strict conformity with the opinions of the majority of the physicians of the Faculté de Médecine, otherwise the thesis was sure to be rejected, as illustrated by the following episode related by Patin in a letter to Charles Spon (December 24, 1655):

A young doctor of the antimonial cabal presented a thesis to the Faculté with this conclusion, *Ergo plueritidis initio purgatio,* which was signed and approved by the Dean *et ipso stibiale.* The Censor of the Faculty opposed the thesis. The Dean, on the contrary judged it would injure his dignity to yield (to the opposition) and ordered the Beadle to distribute (the thesis). The Censor went to see M. Riolan, as the ancient of the College, in order that by his authority he would assemble the company (Faculty), and this he ordered. The Dean named de Bourges, learned the design of M. Riolan, of the Censor, M. le Compte, and of most of the elders, to hold this assembly, where we had about sixty doctors. Guénault even came in order to sustain the thesis. He and his antimonial cabal were shorn. Forty-five of us voted that the thesis should be condemned and revoked, and we ordered the doctor to write another, which shall be approved by the Dean, distributed to the doctors, disputed in due time and place in the College. Meanwhile there is to be a suspension of all acts in the College. The thesis was condemned not as problematic, but as false and criminal, pernicious to the lives of men and to the public welfare.

An unconscious testimony of the importance attached to learning from books instead of reading in the book of nature is given in the following extract from a letter of Patin[2]: "The fourth of May the examination in botany was held in our colleges. Bon Dieu, but they put good questions! One could make a good book of them. There was a doctor who proposed beautiful things, *et plus quam miribilia, de fungis*. It is necessary to have read many books to get from them such a great quantity of good things."

[2] Letter to Charles Spon, June 18, 1658.

Guy Patin's first *thèse quodlibétaire* sustained December 19, 1624, had for its title "Estne feminae in virum mutatio a ἀδύνατος?" which he wisely decided in the negative. On November 27, 1625, he took the negative side in a thesis having for its proposition "An praegnanti periculosè laboranti abortus?"

On March 26, 1626, for his cardinal thesis he chose for his subject "Daturne certum graviditatis indicium ex urina?" again taking the negative side. Pierre Pic[3] remarks that contrary to the usual practice Guy concludes for the negative in each of his three theses and speculates whether this was not an indication of his character, which was already contradictory.

The first thesis at which Patin presided was that of G. Joudounyn, December 16, 1627, entitled "Utrum μηνομανια balneum?" (Are baths useful in uteromania?). Patin is said to have suggested the subject to Joudouyn because of the case of a young girl whom he had attended and whom it is said her mother wished him to marry.[4]

At first the theses were written and presented in manuscript to the Dean of the

[3] Guy Patin, Paris, 1911.

[4] Letter to Falconet, September 19, 1659.

Faculté de Médecine, but toward the end of the sixteenth century the students began to have them printed and as we all know the custom of printing the theses for the doctorate has continued to the present time in France.

After two years passed in this manner, the bachelors presented themselves for examination for the licentiate. Each candidate had to present himself before the docteurs-régents of the Faculté, at the doctor's home, where he was privately examined by that worthy. Then the Faculté would hold a meeting at which a secret ballot was cast by its members, as to whether the candidate should be licensed. If successful he did not at once receive the full license but was first admitted to the ranks of the licentiandes. These happy ones formed a procession and preceded by the beadles of the Faculté, rendered a ceremonial visit to the official bodies in Paris, that is to the members of the Parlement of Paris, the ministers of state, the provost of the merchants and the aldermen, requesting their presence at the solemn ceremony which marked the actual bestowal of the license on those who had passed their examinations. This ceremony of the "Paranymph" derived its name from the ancient Greek marriage custom in which a young man, the best man of the bridegroom, always conducted the latter to the residence of the newly-wedded pair. In this ceremony of the Faculté, the bridegroom was the licentiate, the bride, the Faculté de Médecine and the paranymph was the Dean who united the licentiate in solemn wedlock to the Faculté de Médecine. Some days later there was another grand ceremony in the hall of the Archbishop's palace in Paris, at which the Chancellor of the Faculté de Médecine, who was a canon of the Archdiocese of Paris, gave them the benediction of the church, and afterwards all those present assisted at a grand mass of Notre Dame.

After having become a licentiate, the young man was authorized to practice and teach medicine, but in order to obtain a vote in the deliberations of the Faculté it was necessary for him to go yet further and secure the degree of Doctor of Medicine. This required a further investigation into the learning and morals of the candidate and he had to sustain another thesis, the *vesperie*. Two doctors of the Faculté propounded a question to be discussed by the candidate with them. If he passed this ordeal successfully, the last act of his career as a medical student took place in the grand hall of the École de Médecine, when he received the square bonnet worn by the doctors of the Faculté.

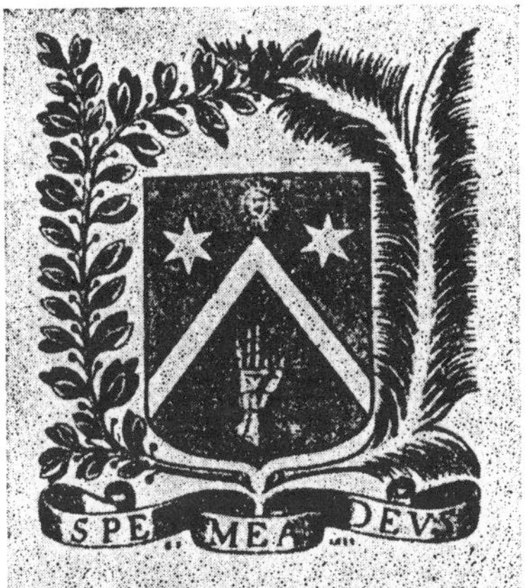

LES ARMES DE GUY PATIN

CHAPTER III

La Faculté de Médecine

To be a member of the Faculté de Médecine de Paris was to Guy the *ne plus ultra* in human affairs. The jealousy with which he guarded the prerogatives of its members was manifested from the time when he first was admitted to its ranks. In Patin's time the question of precedence loomed large in daily life and gave rise to innumerable squabbles. He tells Falconet (November 5, 1649) of one in which he was engaged early in his professional career:

I remember twenty-three years ago, being a young doctor and not yet married, I was asked to carry the canopy (*le ciel*) in a procession of the Holy Sacrement, the day of the grand-fête, which they celebrate here with all sorts of solemnities. I knew about how much I should be esteemed and also how my colleagues had acted in a like case. Being by them incited to do this I promised them I would on condition that because of my rank of docteur-régent of the Faculté, I should have the first place, not ceding it to any but counsellors of the sovereign court. This was promised me, but when I came to take it, with my scarlet cape, as we are clad when we become doctors (receive the degree), dispute, or preside (at meetings) or when we attend the funeral of one of our colleagues, two men wished to have the first place before me, of which one was *conseiller aux monnaies*, the other *secrétaire du roi*. I alleged that it was due me. All the notables of the parish who were gathered for the procession, assembled at once, among them old M. Seguin, *premier médecin de la reine*, who died Dean of our company, January 27, 1648, and said in my favor that I was as great a doctor as he in our Faculté and in Paris. There was also a counsellor of the court, some masters of accounts, and an old advocate, who awarded me the precedence. Those who lost against me gave way at once, out of respect, they said, for the procession, but they grumbled that I should precede them.[1]

[1] Voltaire in "Le siècle de Louis XIV," speaking of the spirit of discord which prevailed in France at the end of the reign of Louis XIII, says that it prevailed throughout the kingdom, extending from the court and Paris to the smallest communes and parishes, in which processions fought one another for the honor of their banners. Often the canons of Notre Dame came to actual fisticuffs with those of Sainte-Chapelle. The Parlement of Paris and the Chambre des Comptes fought one another for precedence actually inside the church of Notre Dame the day that Louis XIII placed his kingdom under the protection of the Virgin Mary, August 5, 1638.

In order to form a just conception of Guy Patin's life and letters some knowledge of the institution about which his whole being centered and which absorbed the greatest part of his energies is absolutely essential. The life interest of Patin was centered in the Faculté de Médecine de Paris. Many men devote their lives to a cause, some to a person and not a few to an institution. The latter was avowedly and definitely the case with Patin. From first to last in almost all of the numerous letters which have been preserved to us, he refers to it or to matters connected with it. The preservation of its rights and privileges, the admission of only those whom he considered worthy to its ranks, the expulsion of those who had proved themselves unworthy of its fellowship, the election of suitable officers to guide its policies, the increase of its authority and wealth and the extension of its usefulness, occupied his mind almost as an obsession. No praise was too fulsome for those who furthered its cause and no abuse too savage for those who dared to attack it. As many of its peculiar attributes brought the Faculté into relation with public men and matters, a very general interest is attached to the life and letters of Patin from the light thrown by them on various political, economic, and social concerns in France during his lifetime. His letters, in addition to their personal characteristics afford a mine of information to the student of French social history during the seventeenth century. The teaching of medicine at Paris was for a long time in the hands of the ecclesiastics, and there was no distinct Faculté or Collège for that purpose at the University of Paris until 1281. From that date the École or Faculté de Médecine forms an entity, and had its own corporate existence in the university body.

Wickersheimer[2] in his most interesting book on the history of medicine in France in the sixteenth century writes of the changes of location the college underwent as it grew in importance with the increase of its students, and gradually eclipsed its ancient rival, the Medical School of Montpellier. At the present time all that remains to recall its former locality to those who search for its traces is to be found in the names still retained by some of the small streets remaining on the left

[2] La médecine et les médecins en France à l'époque de la Renaissance, Paris, 1916.

bank of the Seine, near the Pont St. Michel, the rue de La Bûcherie, the rue de Fouarre, etc., the latter so called from the straw on which the students used to sit. Yet the grand buildings of the present Medical School and its adjuncts are in the immediate neighborhood, and in walking through the rue des Écoles or some of the other new streets, we can realize that for eight hundred years the region has been the home of successive generations of medical teachers and students, and some of the old buildings, such as the church of Saint Severin or the church of Saint Julien-le-Pauvre, though in such a changed environment, remain as monuments of the historic past. In former times religious observances formed a prominent part in the life of the medical school at Paris. It was preeminently Catholic, losing no opportunity to express its devotion to the Faith, expelling from its ranks those suspected of heresy, and during the wars of the League recognizing, under the name of Charles x, the old Cardinal of Bourbon as King of France in opposition to Henri iv. There were many church services which both teachers and students were bound to attend.

The term, Faculté de Médecine, did not imply a few professors or teachers of medicine, but a corporate body of physicians under the control of which was placed the medical teaching of the University, and the control of the practice of medicine in the city of Paris. There were similar faculties elsewhere in France, at Montpellier, Bordeaux, Toulouse, Orleans, Bourges, and many other cities, all possessing locally the same privileges as regarded the exercise of their profession.

The most aged member of the Faculté, known as the Ancient, became solely by nature of his age, an object of respectful veneration on the part of his colleagues. He received double the usual amount of fees or honoraria due to members of the Faculté on the occasion of examinations or other functions, and in case of the incapacity of the Dean from any cause, the Ancient had the right to convoke an assembly of the doctors. The executive chief of the Faculté was the Doyen or Dean, elected for a term of two years. This was a busy and important position. Besides presiding at the meetings of the Faculté, he was present at examinations of students for the various degrees and the readings of the theses. The Dean likewise presided at the examination of those who presented themselves for the right to practice as surgeons and apothecaries, over both of which bodies the Faculté de Médecine had control. He inspected at intervals the shops of all the apothecaries in Paris to ascertain that they obeyed the laws regulating their traffic and that the drugs they kept and sold were pure. He had control of the financial affairs of the Faculté, was the guardian of its seal, and especially of its interests when the Parlement of Paris or any other court or power attempted to infringe upon its rights. As Dean he was one of the governing body of the University and a member of the Parlement of Paris.

Upon the death of a King of France the Ancient and the Dean were both required to attend the autopsy on the defunct, and likewise his funeral, clad in their official robes of scarlet with caps of the same color.

The title of docteur-régent, which Littré in his dictionary says applied to one who instructed publicly, appertained to all members of the Faculté, and until 1505 the function of teaching was performed by any member who felt called upon to do so. In 1505 two teaching chairs were established, and thenceforth many of the docteurs-régents never actually taught classes, although the professors only held the chairs for two years at a time and all members of the Faculté were eligible for election if they desired to become candidates. All the docteurs-régents continued to take part in the examinations and readings of the theses.

The greatest honor which could befall a physician of the Faculté de Médecine de Paris was to be elected its Dean, and this honor fell to the lot of Patin on two occasions, it being practically the invariable custom to re-elect a Dean at the end of his first term. Although Patin, in the years before the choice fell on him, assumes to belittle the position and pretends that it is an honor which he does not desire, it is easy to see from the change in his tone, after elevation to the position, that it had long been an object of ambition for him.

In a letter to Spon (November 24, 1642) Patin relates how near he came to being chosen. The election of a dean was quite a complicated affair. One was held every two years, on the first Saturday after All Saints' Day. The Faculté met in solemn conclave. The Dean whose term was ending read a report of the period during which he had held office. The names of all the doctors present were then written on separate ballots, and those of the junior doctors deposited in one urn, and those of the senior doctors in another. The Dean shook the ballots up and then drew two from among the juniors, and three from among the seniors. The five doctors thus chosen by lot took an oath to designate the most worthy for the position of Dean. They retired to the Chapel, where they chose three names by a majority vote, two seniors and one junior. Three tickets bearing these names were placed in a hat and the Dean drew one of them from it, and the happy owner of it became Dean for the ensuing two years. Patin tells Spon that his name "danced in the hat" with those of Messieurs Perreau and de la Vigne but that "the lot is always contrary to me," and Monsieur de la Vigne won the election. Writing to Belin, *fils*,[3] (November 16, 1652) Patin says that he has sent him the jeton, or medal, struck by order of the Faculté in honor of his decanate. These jetons were always struck to com-

[3] The Belins, with whom Patin corresponded, were a father and son each named Claude who practiced medicine at Troyes, where there were also several other physicians of the same family. Their names are preserved solely in the correspondence of Patin.

memorate the elevation of a Dean of the Faculty. In the ANNALS OF MEDICAL HISTORY[4] a number of them including that of Patin, are reproduced from the numismatic collection of the Army Medical Library at Washington, with a most interesting description of them by Dr. Albert Alleman.

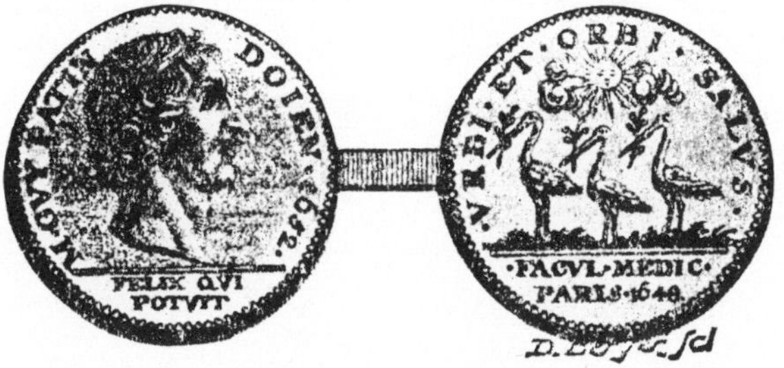

Jeton of Guy Patin

Patin writes to Falconet (June 28, 1652):

The custom is to put the arms of the Dean on one side and those of the Faculté on the other. I have retained the latter, but instead of putting those of my family which are gules with a gold chevron, accompanied by two gold stars *en chef*, and a hand pointing in gold, I have put my portrait. The engraver, skilful as he is, has not caught the resemblance very well, especially the eye, but there is no remedy.

Patin's greatest object in life was the preservation and if possible extension of

[4] New York, 1917. I, ii, 156,157.

the privileges and authority of the Faculté de Médecine de Paris. Page after page of his correspondence is devoted to this theme and he constantly speaks with pride, in his letters to the Belins at Troyes, to Spon at Lyons, or to other doctors in the provinces, of the glory of the Faculté and of the proofs which it gives from time to time of its strength in its various contests with the apothecaries, the surgeons or other enemies who strove to encroach on its prerogatives. Thus he writes in February, 1558, that he has seen in the coffers of the Faculté, a royal decree entitled "Nouvelle confirmation de l'an 1132." He adds a disquisition on the powers possessed by the Dean, he is "the master of the schools, he has all the keys; fourteen handsome registers, all the records, and all the money, of which he renders an exact account every year, he is *vindex disciplinae et custos legum.* Our statutes call him *caput Facultatis.*"

He consoles himself for his defeat, by the reflection that the honor is accompanied by "a very heavy and very difficult responsibility." Writing to Falconet (November 4, 1650) he says: "I have been an elector many times, I have even been chosen and put in the hat three times, and each of the three I have remained at the bottom of the hat, and if ever they put me in it again, I shall not be vexed to remain there."

The lot finally proved favorable to Patin and on November 5, 1650, he was elected Dean. Although he affects to speak somewhat deprecatingly at times, saying, "I have already enough business without this," nevertheless much more frequently his pride in the position pours forth. On December 1, 1650, he gave the customary banquet to the members of the Faculté, and he writes to Falconet the next day that thirty-six of his colleagues had enjoyed his hospitality:

I never saw so much laughing and drinking by serious men, and even our ancients; it was the best wine of Bordeaux which I had chosen for the feast. I entertained them in my chamber where over the hangings were displayed the pictures of Erasmus, the two Scaligers, father and son, Casaubon, Muret, Montaigne, Charron, Grotius, Heinsius, Saumaise, Fernel, de Thou, and our good friend M. G. Naudé, librarian for Mazarin . . . there were yet three other portraits of excellent men, of the late M. de Sales, bishop of Geneva, M., the bishop de Bellay, my good friend; Justus Lipsius, and finally François Rabelais, for which one has offered to give me twenty pistoles. What say you to this assemblage? Were not my guests in good company?

Writing to Spon (March 6, 1656):

When I shall receive your picture I will put it in a good place with Fernel, Ellain, Duport, Seguin, Marescot, Nicolas Pietre, the late M. Riolan, André du Laurens, the late M. Gassendi, Salmasius, Heinsius, Grotius, Naudaeus, Muret, Buchanan, the two Scaligers, Lipsius, Thuanus (de Thou), Crassot, Passerat, Campanella, Fra Paolo Sarpi, Casaubon, the Chancellor de l'Hôpital, P. Charron, Michel de Montaigne; the French author otherwise named Rabelais, the divine Erasmus, etc.[5]

In the letter quoted above, writing to Belin, *fils* (January 14, 1651) Patin says:

I should tell you that our Faculté made me Dean the fifth of last November, a charge to which I had been elected and named four other times; it is difficult and takes much time, but it is honorable. . . . My wife says there is much good fortune for the end of the year, her husband, Dean, her eldest son, doctor, and a good house which she greatly wished for.

[5] Pic publishes as an addendum to his Guy Patin the pictures of all those who figured in Patin's gallery.

Patin's pride in the Faculté de Médecine is well expressed in a letter[6] in which he says:

All individual men die, but associations do not die. The most powerful man in the last one hundred years in Europe without being a crowned head, was the Cardinal Richelieu. He made the whole earth tremble, he caused terror at Rome; he treated rudely and shook the King of Spain, and nevertheless he was not able to make us receive into our company the two sons of the Gazetteer (Renaudot) who were licensed but who will not be doctors for a long time.

No one could have had a higher idea of the powers of the Dean than Patin and once, at least, he got himself into trouble by an undue exercise of them. Doctor Pic gives the story with some additional information supplied by the researches of his friend, M. Delalain. Jean Chartier, a docteur-régent, published without the approval of the Faculté de Médecine, a book on antimony. Patin removed his name from the list of docteurs-régents, and Chartier appealed to Parlement for reinstatement. The court of the Parlement rendered its

[6] Letter to Spon, December 6, 1644.

judgment, July 15, 1653, in favor of Chartier and ordered that he should be reinstated as docteur-régent; that Patin should pay him 48 livres parisis in amend, all the expenses of his reinstatement, and two-thirds of the costs of the trial, the other one-third to be paid by the other docteurs-régents, Germain Hureau and Daniel Arbinet, who had acted with Patin in the matter; and these three were enjoined from any act or word interfering with Chartier in the future enjoyment of the rights and privileges of his position in the Faculté de Médecine.

He tells Belin he has a copy of all the names and surnames of the licentiates and doctors according to their order of passing at the École de Paris for more than three centuries, with all the memorable events in the Faculté. In a letter to Belin, *fils* (January, 1651) he tells of a book written by M. Moreau, "De antiquitate facultatis medicae Parisiensis," which is not yet published and he fears will not be because of the ill health of Moreau, but which would be very curious and beautiful. He tried to secure all the biographical details possible about the lives of those who had been physicians at Paris. He writes to Spon (December 30, 1650): "There is scarcely a bachelor or a licentiate, much less a doctor of our schools for upward of three hundred years of whom I cannot tell something, even if only a little."

In a letter of the same date (December 30, 1650) to Falconet he tells him how he had recovered some of the old registers of the Faculté which had disappeared:

An honest friend of mine, knowing that I had been elected Dean of our Faculté in the place of M. Jean Pietre, the 5th of last November, has placed in my hands an old register of our Schools, in abridged characters almost Gothic, from the year 1390, in which is noted every two years the number of doctors and of licentiates.

Those of the doctors are sometimes fifteen, twenty, twenty-five, going even to forty. I lent it to M. Riolan who found in it the mention of an honest man who left by will a manuscript of Galen which he had, *de usu partium.* This legacy dates from the year 1009, and is of further consequence because it proves against those who would doubt it, that in that year and before it, there was a Faculté de Médecine at Paris.

A curious feature in the medical life of the seventeenth century can be found in a study of the family relationship which prevailed among the great men of the profession, constituting veritable dynasties, in whose hands were held the great preferments and choicest clientele. The Riolans, Pietres, Moreaus, Seguins and many others might be adduced as interesting instances.

Jean Riolan, the elder, transmitted his fame and position to his son, Jean. The elder Riolan's wife was Anne Pietre, daughter of the first Simon Pietre. Charles Bouvard, first physician to Louis XIII and superintendent of the Jardin des Plantes, was a brother-in-law of Riolan, and Bouvard's daughter married Jacques Cousinot, first physician to Louis XIV. Thus it will be seen that Bouvard, the Riolans and Cousinot were connected with the Pietres, the most prominent medical family in Paris for a period of many years. The first of the family of Pietre to become prominent in medical affairs was Simon Pietre (1525–1584). He was a Huguenot, and his life was saved during the Massacre of St. Bartholomew by his son-in-law, Riolan, who concealed him in the abbey of St. Victor. In spite of his religion he was made physician to Charles IX by Catherine de' Medici. Curiously, Ambroise Paré, also accused of Huguenotism (perhaps secretly

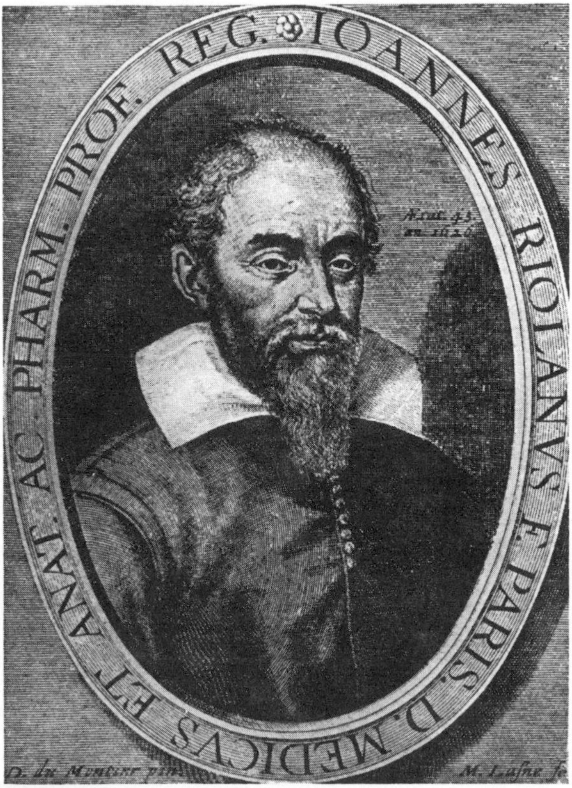

JEAN RIOLAN, THE YOUNGER
(1577–1657)

a Huguenot) was also favored by Catherine and was first surgeon to Charles IX. The first Simon Pietre's son, also named Simon (1565–1618), married the daughter of the celebrated physician Marescot. He succeeded Gourmelen, the infamous enemy of Ambroise Paré, as professor of medicine at the Collège Royal. Another son of old Simon, named Nicolas, was a distinguished physician, and his son Jean had a very large practice and was esteemed a most learned physician. There were five doctors of the same family who figured largely in the medical profession at Paris during the seventeenth century under the name of Akakia, a Greek version of their real family name, Sans-Malice. One of them, Martin Akakia, was a brother-in-law of one of the Seguins and succeeded him as Professeur du Roi at Paris. Patin says that he resigned his chair in 1655, after having held it for many years without daring to give a public lecture.

There were also three or four Moreaus and equal numbers of Seguins who shared or transmitted their various dignities among one another.

Whatever may be thought of the narrowness or ultra-conservatism of the Faculté de Médecine in Patin's time it should in justice be conceded that it attempted to place medical education on a higher plane. Patin writes to Belin (July 29, 1654) that in some cities anyone who claimed to have a medical degree could settle and practice medicine, but in Paris and in other places those who wished to practice had to undergo an examination to ascertain their abilities no matter from whence they had graduated, "and this rigor is not without benefit for the purpose of remedying the abuse which is heaped upon many of the little universities and even upon the larger ones that sometimes give doctors' degrees too easily for money."

In spite of the fact that Patin never became, in the strict sense of the term, one of the physicians to the court, his letters are full of references to medical matters connected with the court, and of tales of those physicians whom the king delighted to honor.

From the tone of many of these, one cannot but feel that there was considerable personal animus and chagrin at his exclusion from their midst, but it is impossible to imagine Guy in the rôle of a courtier, and in the long run perhaps it was as well for his happiness that he did not achieve court distinction. In order that some of the references in his letters may be rendered less obscure, it is as well to pause for a moment to glance at the organization of the court physicians, that we may realize some of the responsibilities and emoluments incumbent on them.

The medical service at the court of France during the seventeenth century was organized on the same lavish scale as all the other services of the Maison du Roi. Positions in it were eagerly sought after and were frequently sold for very high prices. Thus Patin writes Spon (May 3, 1650) that Seguin who had seven years before paid Guillemeau 50,000 livres for the succession to his place as médecin ordinaire du roi, had in turn sold the succession to de la Chambre for 22,000 *écus*, and he writes to Falconet (July 5, 1652) of the death of Vautier:

He (Vautier) was premier médecin du roi and the last of the kingdom in capacity, and in order that you should know that he is not dead without cause, he took antimony thrice, that he might die in his method, by the consent and advice of Guénault. If he had died seven years ago he would have saved the lives of many honest men who have been killed by his antimony. At length he is dead himself aged fifty-three years. As he was reported to be very ignorant even at Court he wished to have the reputation of possessing chemical secrets and of excelling in the preparation of antimony. Some courtiers applauded him or seemed to do so. The authority of his charge sustained his credit. He said among other things that the physicians of Paris were right to say that antimony was a poison, but that as he prepared it, it was not; nevertheless this good preparation failed him. It is a place vacant for which Cardinal Mazarin expects (*cherche*) three thousand pistoles, there is one of my colleagues who says that they have offered it to Guénault at that price, but that he refused it, but that he believes that Valot will give them. Thus all is for sale, even to the health of the king which is a very bad example.

At the head of the medical service there was the premier médecin, the first physician to the king. He was one of the grand officers of the crown, a member of the council of state, and ennobled by virtue of his position, bearing a coat of arms. He received a large salary and many perquisites, such as we know Fernel, physician to Henri II received at the birth of each of the children of his royal master. Of course, in consequence of his office, he was sure of a large clientele among the nobility. He had authority over all the physicians, surgeons, apothecaries, dentists, etc., who aided him in guarding the health of the royal person, judging as to their qualifications for their respective appointments, and assuring himself that they fulfilled their duties properly. He was required to be in attendance each morning when the king arose, and to exercise an active supervision over the king's diet and regimen. If the king was ill the first physician had chief care of the case and direction of its management, presiding at all consultations and carefully observing the results of the medicines or remedies administered to him. It was his duty to accompany the king on any journey he might make, and he had to take up his residence at whatever château or place the court might lodge.

Associated with him were eight physicians in ordinary, or as they were generally termed, physicians by quarter, because of the division of their terms of service in attendance by quarters of the year. Two of them were required to be in attendance at the court for three months in each year. During that time they slept near the king, attended the rising and retirement of the king, and were present at his meals. The constant supervision of the meat and drink of the king was necessary not only in order to see that it was properly prepared, but also to guard against the danger of an attempt to poison the monarch.

There were many instances of the appointment of additional physicians to the king. These received their appointments generally by their successful management of some patient belonging to the royal family, rarely because of any especially distinguished standing in the profession. Undoubtedly many of the court physicians owed their positions to some lucky chance or to the backing of influential friends, while on the other hand, many were appointed because by their merit they had obtained a reputation for skill. Thus Ambroise Paré's appointment as chief surgeon was due to the recognition of his skill by those whom he had treated in the wars.

Patin tells Belin (October 28, 1631) that Senelles, one of the king's physicians, had been tried for casting a horoscope of the king and predicting his death. He and another of the king's physicians, Duval, who was concerned with him in the matter, were sentenced to the galleys for life and their property confiscated.

Again writing to him in 1655, he says that Louis XIV is ill at Fontainebleau with a continued fever, he has been bled from the arms and one foot. The fever developed after he had been taken by his physicians to drink the waters at Forges.

God knows for what reason they should make a young prince of seventeen years drink those lye waters when in as good a state of health as was the king. It has been long that princes have been unfortunate in their physicians. I wish with all my heart that God sends him good health, and that they do not give him antimony. Note that in all the court there is not a good physician.

Writing again (March 14, 1657) he reiterates his views:

The great are unfortunate in their physicians. The chief number of the court physicians are ignorant or charlatans, and often both the one and other.

The premier chirurgien or first surgeon to the king, was assisted by eight surgeons in ordinary, or by quarter. His office was subordinate to that of the premier médecin, and his duties not quite so onerous.

The court physician had no easy task. Louis XIV would not let Fagon use the word "order" (*ordonnance*) when prescribing for him, and Louis xv reprimanded his physician when he told him "it was necessary" (*il faut*) that he should do or take something. When Senac was appointed médecin du roi in 1752, he had Fizes appointed to the position of physician to the duc d'Orléans which he had previously held. Senac gave Fizes some advice as to the behavior he should adopt towards his noble patient:

I told him to approach his patient gravely, to feel his pulse, make him put out his tongue, gaze seriously in the basin (urinal or else bowl in which the blood had been drawn); not to speak, but to shroud himself in his peruke, and remain thus a moment with his eyes closed, then to give his orders, and go away without thinking to make his reverence. Instead of that, my imbecile jabbered like a magpie; he talked politics and literature, saying, "Your serene highness" every minute. He only got what he merited, and that is what should happen to all those who do not listen to their elders. Fizes was discharged within a month after he had been appointed.

When Louis xiv came to the throne, Cousinot held the position of first physician.

Patin writes Charles Spon (December 6, 1644) about the intrigues which were on foot to secure the position for Vautier. The latter had been physician to Marie de' Medici. In 1630 he had been sent to the Bastille where he had remained for twelve years, probably because of participation in the intrigues of the Queen Mother. In 1644 he was physician-in-ordinary to Cardinal Mazarin. Patin writes that Cardinal Richelieu had never dared put his physician, Citois, in the position of physician to the King, fearing that it would rouse suspicions against him. He thinks that for that reason, if for no other Vautier would never receive the appointment. Also Anne of Austria, the Queen Mother, who was regent for Louis XIV, esteemed Cousinot and did not wish to have him ousted. Vautier ultimately received the appointment of first physician to Louis XIV. Patin writes Spon (May 29, 1648) that Vautier had complained to a friend of his that he was dissatisfied with his income and wished to obtain another benefice. The friend pointed out to Vautier that he should be content as he received 25,000 *écus* from this position, besides what he made from his practice at Court, and the revenue he received from an abbey, and that having already this benefice he should not seek to obtain further revenues from the Church. Vautier replied that he did not feel his conscience charged nor his soul in danger for the benefice he held and that he would not be damned any quicker for three abbeys than for one.

Mazarin had had his favorite Valot appointed médecin du roi, when the King was sick with a malarial fever, or possibly typhoid. Patin writes Spon (October 19, 1655):

The Queen has refused Valot permission to bring physicians to Fontainebleau to consult with him, and treat the king. He had named A. Daquin and Veson to her. She answered in anger: "I doubt the choice which you would make. These are fine physicians for the King! I do not agree with you. I wish to have Guénault who treated him once when he had smallpox." Guénault was sent for and is there. One holds that Valot is in danger of being discharged, although he has not yet touched any money since the three years that he payed to enter there; at least he is in great danger of it if the Cardinal does not maintain him and put him back in the good graces of the King and Queen, with whom he stands very badly.

A few days later Patin writes that he had been at a consultation with Riolan and Moreau, in the course of which they had told him that the King had called Valot an ignoramus and charlatan and the Queen had treated him with great rudeness but that Mazarin backed him up. Sometime before the King's illness a son of Valot's had died and Valot had asked the King to bestow a benefice which he had held on another of his sons, but the King had refused. The Queen sent for Guénault to come and see the King but Mazarin sent him back to Paris. A little later, in November, Patin tells Spon that Mazarin has abandoned the cause of Valot, in turn calling him an ignoramus and a charlatan and saying that he was the cause of the King's illness.

Molière's epigram on the death of Henrietta Maria, the Queen of England, sister of Louis XIII, under the care of Valot might be recalled:

> Le croiriez vous, race future,
> Que la fille du grand Henri
> Eut en mourant même aventure
> Que fut son père et son mari?
> Tous trois sont morts par assasin,
> Ravaillac, Cromwell, médecin;
> Henri, d'un coup de baionette,
> Charles fini sur son billot,
> Et maintenant meure Henriette,
> Par l'ignorance de Valot.

On March 23, 1663, Patin in a long letter to Falconet sums up a great deal of information about the court physicians of his time, getting his knowledge from a book which Bouvard had written and proposed to publish. Before doing so he had submitted copies of the manuscript to Moreau and Patin and to his father-in-law, Riolan. The latter advised Moreau not to publish the book as he would incur the enmity not only of Valot and Vautier but also of Cardinal Mazarin. Bouvard thereupon got Moreau and Patin to give him back the manuscripts he had submitted to them. Patin quotes his recollections of what Bouvard had written and of conversations he had had with him on the subject of the court physicians. Bouvard told him that once he had talked to Louis XIII about Héroard, Guillemeau and Vautier and that the King had said: "I, also, am unfortunate to have been in the hands of so many charlatans." Héroard was a good courtier with a thirst for riches. He got enmeshed in the troubles of the Queen Mother, Marie de' Medici, and Richelieu stopped his further progress at the Court. Vautier was a miserable Jew of Avignon, very boastful and ignorant. He was the physician and friend of the Queen Mother and was implicated with the Marillacs in their designs against Richelieu.

On the famous Journée des Dupes, November 11, 1630, when Richelieu overthrew their conspiracy, Vautier was arrested and passed nearly twelve years in the Bastille. When Mazarin came into power during the regency of Anne of Austria, Vautier was appointed first physician to the King. Patin says that this same Vautier was used by Mazarin as a spy at the Court.

CHAPTER IV

Home Life and Literary Interests

HOME LIFE

Patin soon achieved sufficient practice to give him a very comfortable position in life. He speaks with pardonable pride of his possessions. Writing to Belin (May 1, 1630) he says: "I have in this city two things of which I can boast, good books and good friends, which are at your service." And again writing to Belin, *fils*, in January, 1651, he states:

> Furthermore I have purchased a fine house, in which I have dwelt now for three days. It is situated in the Place du Chevalier du Guet, *en belle vue*, and away from noise. . . . I have a fine, large, vast study in which I hope to place my 10,000 books by adding to it a little chamber which is on the same floor. My friends say I am the best lodged man in Paris.

He writes to both Spon and Falconet about his removal to his new house but dwells chiefly on the pleasure it gives him to have his books so well lodged. He describes the arrangement of his study in a letter to Falconet (April 24, 1651):

I assure you it is beautiful. I have put on the mantle of the chimney a beautiful picture of a crucifix which a painter that I had had cut (for stone) had given me in 1627. On either side of the good God are both of us, the master and the mistress; under the crucifix are the portraits of Erasmus and J. Scaliger. . . . Besides the ornaments which are on my chimney, there is in the middle of my library a large beam, which passes from one end to the other on each side of which there are a dozen pictures of illustrious men, having thus plenty of light from the opposite windows, so that I am in good company with good illumination.

He writes of his method of moving his books,[1] "All my folios are moved and arranged in their places, there are already more than sixteen hundred in order. We have commenced to move the quartos after which will follow the octavos, and thus to the end of the procession which will last yet a month."

No wonder such a booklover could write his friend Spon (August, 1658) seven years later: "I hold myself more fortunate at home with my books and a little leisure,

[1] Letter to Charles Spon, January, 1651.

than Mazarin with all his *écus* and inquietudes."

Patin evidently enjoyed comparing his state with that of the detested Mazarin, for he writes Falconet (February 28, 1650) that he had been told on good authority that Mazarin thought of going into retirement, adding that, however that might be, "I esteem myself a thousand times happier than he, being enclosed in good company with my silent masters, while I hear the dancing and violins at my neighbors who are rejoicing in the carnival and would not believe it was carême if they did not play the fool all these days of feasting."

Some years later he gives Falconet (November 8, 1658) a pleasant picture of the way he spent his evenings with his two illustrious neighbors, M. Miron, *président aux enquêtes* and M. Charpentier, *conseiller aux requêtes:*

Our conversation is always gay. If we talk of religion or of the State it is only historically without dreaming of reformation or sedition. We talk to one another about things as they are. Our principal conversation regards literature, of that which is new, worth consideration and useful. The mind thus refreshed I return to my house, where after some intercourse with my books, or an urgent consultation, I seek sleep in my bed, which is without falsehood, as said our grand Fernel, according to the tragic Seneca, *pars humanae melior*. I seldom sup out of my house, only occasionally, with M. de Lamoignon, premier president.

The book-lover Patin complains to Belin (September, 1646) that it has been necessary for him to make three journeys from Paris, one into Beauce, one to Rouen, and another into Normandy:

However-so-much I love the sedentary life and not to go away from Paris, because of my books. If I did not know myself well I would say of myself what an old surgeon of Paris said of himself "that he was persecuted by too much practice because he was too skilful a man." . . . These journeys were as displeasing to me as they were necessary for those for whom I made them, and they moreover were extremely incommoding to me.

There is no indication that Patin ever left his beloved Paris for any length of time. He writes to Charles Spon (March 13, 1648) about a projected journey on which he proposed to go first to Lyons to visit him, thence to Geneva, from there to Bâle, to visit the famous anatomist Bauhin and the tomb of the great Erasmus. Then he proposed to go to Nuremberg, where Volckamer would introduce him to Gaspard Hoffmann. In returning he would visit his brother at Nimegue and some of the cities of Holland, to wit; the Hague, Leiden, Amsterdam, Rotterdam, and Dordrecht. At Rotterdam he would seek out the birthplace of the "incomparable Erasmus" and at Leiden he wished to visit with devout respect the tomb of the "very great man, Joseph Scaliger." His eldest son, Robert, was to accompany him on the trip. For some reason, probably the uncertain state of the various countries through which he would travel, the plan was given up.

In a letter to Spon (June 13, 1644) Patin says that five years after receiving his doctor's degree he took a wife "from whom I will have in direct succession 20,000 *écus*, her father and mother yet living but very old, with one collateral (relative) a sister who has no children and is very rich. God has blessed my alliance with four sons, to wit Robert, Charles, Pierrot and François."

Patin also owned a county house of which he wrote Belin, *fils*, July 5, 1651: "My wife and children are in the country at three leagues from here, in a handsome house, which I bought for fifteen thousand livres."

LITERARY INTERESTS

Patin's intense interest in the history and literature of his profession is manifest throughout all his life. He begins his correspondence with Belin (in 1630, aged twenty-nine) by telling him that he is trying to make a collection of all the theses read at the medical school in Paris and asks him for copies of those which he could not obtain at Paris and thought Belin might have at Troyes, written by Belin's contemporaries at Paris.

Patin had also the most lively interest in general literature. In 1637 there was published an edition of the Latin addresses pronounced by Jean Passerat, one of the authors of the "Satire Ménippée" and professor of eloquence and Latin poetry in the Collège Royal, with a preface by Guy Patin. In addition to writing to his friends the news about all the latest medical books and editions, he writes of works on law, theology, philosophy, literature and history, rejoicing in new editions of Vossius, Lipsius, Casaubon, Scaliger, Grotius, etc.

Patin was a veritable bibliomaniac and occasionally his conscience seems to have smitten him for the constant importunities with which he beset his friends. Thus he writes[2] to one of them: "Pardon me the many importunities which I make to you because of my bibliomania, it is a sickness of which I cannot cure myself this year; perhaps I will amend next year."

He also admits that his studious habits injured his health. He says[3]: "I occupy myself so much with my books, of which I purchase a new one nearly every day, that I pass with them all the day and the night, but these vigils have injured my health so much, that to reestablish it I have had to almost abandon my studies. This is one of the obligations that I owe to medicine, without the succour of which I would undoubtedly have killed myself in my desire to become too learned."

In 1668 Patin published the "Apologia pro Galeno," written by Gaspard Hoffmann, who died in 1648. Patin purchased the manuscript after Hoffmann's death. He dedicated the book to his friend, President Lamoignon.

[2] Letter to Charles Spon, January 11, 1655.

[3] Letter to Falconet, September 19, 1659.

Patin not only collected and read books but he was an active factor in stimulating the publication of new works and of new editions of those which were difficult to obtain or which in his opinion were suitable for republication in improved form. With this object in view he was constantly importing books from Holland, Germany or Italy, lending rare manuscripts or tomes to publishers, and writing to procure such material from sources where he thought it might be obtained. And his zeal extended to other fields than those of his profession. Thus we find him writing (April 1, 1657) to M. de Tournes, a bookseller, offering his aid in publishing various books. Writing to Belin (August 2, 1640): "If ever you come across the Volume of Epistles by Erasmus in folio, the thickness of three big fingers (because there are others that are smaller), purchase it boldly; it is a book worth its weight in gold." Patin contemplated getting out a work on practice of his own, a "Methodus" or manual, and wrote to Spon (July 13, 1649) about the plan he proposed to follow, but which he never carried out.

In writing to Belin (November 4, 1631) Patin, speaking of the last edition of Paré's works, says: "The Paré of the last impression, well bound, costs eight livres, without any rebate. It is augmented in this last (edition) by a new treatise on fevers, which has been added at the end of the book, and is written by a physician *intus et in cute mihi noto*, without having put his name to it, which is very good." Triaire believes it very probable that the anonymous physician, whose "name was very good" and whom Patin knew so well, was none other than Guy himself.

Writing to Spon (June 11, 1649) Patin after stating that Paré had decried the use of unicorn's horn and other Arabesque remedies, adds: "Do not think of rejecting the opinion of Paré under cover that he was only a surgeon. The author of his book was a learned physician of Paris, named Master Jean Hautin (Altinus), who died here, one of our ancients, in the year 1615." This repeats an accusation made by Le Paulmier, Riolan and others that the works appearing under the name of Paré were not really written by the Father of French surgery, but by others. Malgaigne[4] in the Introduction to his definitive edition of the writings of Paré has proved convincingly the falsity of such statements, and shown

[4] Oeuvres complètes d'Ambroise Paré. Paris, 1840.

beyond cavil that Paré never put forth a line of which he was not the veritable author. Patin possibly was misled by his admiration for Riolan to share the views which the animosity of the latter towards Paré caused him to propagate.

Patin translated into Latin and published with notes the works of André du Laurens (1538–1609), premier physician to Marie de' Medici, and after the death of Marescot, to Henri IV.

RELIGIOUS BELIEF

Patin was not openly a Huguenot but had strong sympathies with them and he was certainly not a very strict Catholic. He read many Huguenot works on theology. He frequently expresses admiration for Arnauld and other Jansenists. Thus he writes Spon (March 3, 1656): "The Jansenists are badly and iniquitously treated by the Sorbonne which I impute to the injustice of the age and the impiety which prevails, and also to the too great power of the Loyolists who are their powerful enemies." Writing to Belin (October 28, 1631) he says: "In our Christian religion I believe as we all should believe, many things that we do not see . . . but it is by means of the faith which obliges us to; . . . but in medicine I believe only that which I see."

He admired the writings of Calvin. In a letter to Falconet (May 24, 1650) he says:

There never was a man as learned as Calvin in ecclesiastical history. At the age of twenty-two he was the most learned man in Europe. I was once at a banquet at one of our graduation exercises where one of our old doctors named Bazin said that Calvin had falsified all the Holy Scriptures. But I took up the good man whom I rendered so ridiculous, that M. Guénault, the younger, who was near me said that I pushed him too much and that I should have pity on his age and debility. Jean de Montluc, bishop of Valence, said that Calvin was the greatest theologian in the world. Have no fear that they say as much in Rome.

On April 10, 1665 he writes to Falconet that "as a good parishioner" he had that morning attended mass at Saint-Germain l'Auxerrois where he saw the King who was present in great state.

Writing to Belin, *fils*, apropos of the Dutch and their wars he says: "But the Pope and the Jesuits will never fail to arouse a war against those men, who will not believe in Purgatory, nor purchase from them indulgences, medals, blessed grains and other spiritual bijoux." He writes several times in 1660 that he is anxiously awaiting a book of Huguenot theses which is being published at Genoa. He also refers several times in the same year to a Latin translation of the Bible made in England with notes by Calvin, Beza, and other Huguenots. Yet he tells Belin (February 7, 1648) that he belongs to the Parish of Saint-Germain-l'Auxerrois and he was interred in that church after his death. He refers sympathetically in several places to the Huguenots massacred in Savoy.

He writes a confession of faith to Belin (July 18, 1642):

I put no credence or belief in possessions, nor in sorcerers, nor miracles that I neither see nor discern. I believe all that is contained in the New Testament, as an article of faith, but I will not give like authority to all the legends of the monks, *fabulosis et commentitiis narrationibus Loyolitarum*, who in the romances which they send us from the Indies, say things as impertinent and as untrue as the fables of Æsop. You would say that these men worked only to infatuate the world. It is true that if we were all wise, these master pharisees of Christianity would be in danger of soon dying of hunger, *Credo in Deum Christum crucifixum, etc. de minimis non curat practor*. Deception, horrible thing, is altogether unworthy of an honest man, but it is even worse when it is mixed in and employed in religious affairs, *Christus ipse, qui veritas est, non indiget mendacio.* I cannot put up with the stinking falsehoods which the monks retail to the world to authorize their cabal, and it astonishes me greatly, *imo serio irascor*, that they have so much credit.

A friend of Spon's who met Patin at Paris thought he was an ecclesiastic. Patin writes to Spon (January 24, 1651):

I pray you to salute M. Sarrazin on my part and tell him that I am much vexed that he should have taken me for a priest, seeing that I am not and never shall be one, and even that I had not wished to be in spite of the efforts of my mother, and that I have often praised God that he did not make me a woman, a priest, a Turk or a Jew.

Tallemant des Reaux[5] relates that Patin, whom he terms a learned physician of the Faculty, pretended that one of his patients when dying had promised to return after his death and tell him if there really was a purgatory. Patin said that the dead man did appear to him one morning, but that

[5] Les historiettes de Tallemant des Reaux, II, 193, Paris, 1840.

he did not speak, because those who return from the other world never talk.

Patin was a great admirer of Jansen and of Arnauld. He speaks of their writings in terms of the highest esteem and condemns in unmitigated terms on many occasions the persecution which they suffered at the hands of the ecclesiastical authorities.

From some of the many references to him in the Letters, it would appear that Patin knew Arnauld, or at any rate had seen him. He describes[6] him as follows: "M. Arnauld is a little, dark, ugly man, born at Paris, the son of a learned advocate, who formerly plead vigorously against the Jesuits . . . He is a doctor of the Sorbonne and very learned, aged forty-six years . . . and one of the most brilliant men of the day."

Patin frequently expresses great admiration for Jean Duvergier de Hauranne, Abbé of Saint-Cyran, who wrote a book in which he belabored the Jesuits. It was entitled "Petrus Aurelius" and was published anonymously in 1653. Amongst other hard things he said the Jesuits were "*Omnium adulatores et omnium inimici*" (The flatterers and enemies of everybody). This phrase Patin frequently quotes with cordial

[6] Letter to Charles Spon, February 26, 1656

approval. The book went through several editions and was warmly approved of by many of the clergy. Godeau, the Bishop of Grasse, especially, wrote in praise of the author. The Jesuits, however, finally succeeded in having it suppressed. Saint-Cyran died of apoplexy in October, 1643, and Patin writes[7] that he was loved and revered by all worthy men and above all at the Sorbonne.

Patin was greatly delighted with the "Provincial Letters" (Lettres Provinciales) of Pascal. They appeared in 1656 and created a great sensation. Their circulation was prohibited, but Guy writes Spon that he will send them to him and tells him what rage and consternation they have created among the Jesuits. Patin writes repeatedly of the massacres of the Protestants of Vaudois, speaking of them as "the poor Huguenots," and stating several times his joy at hearing that Cromwell had interfered on their behalf. He proposed to demand the punishment of those who had instigated and conducted the massacres.

He writes to Spon (January 19, 1656):

The pest is yet very bad at Rome, but it spares the pope and the cardinals. Perhaps it is

[7] Letter to Charles Spon, October 26, 1643.

because it thinks they are more evil than it. Nevertheless thirty-six good and wise physicians are dead, and it is they whom I regret. The pope and the cardinals never lack. There are always enough of them.

Also (November 18, 1659): "If the pest took only monks, generals of orders, and especially the general of the Jesuits, I think Christianity would hardly lose."

Patin's narrative of the so-called "Miracle of Port Royal" is very amusing. A niece of Pascal's suffered from a lachrymal fistula and according to the Port Royalists, was cured by the application of a thorn which had been one of those in the Crown of Thorns. The miraculous cure was certified by four physicians, Bouvard, Hamon, and the two sons of Patin's old enemy, Renaudot. Patin laughs at the whole affair in a letter to Spon (November 7, 1656) saying it was put forth as counterblast to the many miracles claimed by the Jesuits. He adds:

Some have asked me my opinion. I answered it was perhaps a miracle that God had permitted to Port Royal to console those poor people that one calls Jansenists, who for three years have been persecuted by the pope, the Jesuits, the Sorbonne, and the greater part of the deputies of the clergy, also to lower the pride of the Jesuits, who are very insolent and impudent, because of some credit which they have at Court.

Writing to de Salins, a physician at Beaume (March 27, 1655), he tells him to make a little hidden library containing among other lesser known books those of Rabelais, Marot, Montaigne and Erasmus:

Your book by Marot[8] is not bad. Guard it well and hide it for fear the monks steal it from you and burn it. Put with it M. François Rabelais', the Catholicon of Spain (one of the most popular satires against the League). The Republic of Bodin, the Politiques of Lipsius, the Essays of Montaigne, the Sagesse of Charron, the Doctrine curieuse of Père Grasse, the Récherche des récherches, these are books which are capable of taking the world by the nose. I would except from them the two last which are good for other reasons. Do not neglect them and make of them a little library which will be a *reductis et extra insidias monachorum.*

For the writings of Erasmus, keep them, *propter authoris dignitatem.*

[8] Clement-Marot wrote a metrical version of the Psalms in French about the middle of the sixteenth century. It was very popular with the Huguenots and equally hated by the Catholics.

O the excellent man that he was! Drink a little of the good wine of Beaune to his memory, *cum novella uxore*, and I will give you reason on the first occasion. Read his Colloquies once a year and place them in the library above mentioned, *cum ejusdem authoris lingua et encomio moriae atque institutione principis christinae.*

Patin professes a great admiration for the "Religio Medici" of Sir Thomas Browne. In a letter to Spon (October 21, 1644) he writes:

There has arrived here from Holland a little book, entirely new, entitled Religio Medici, written by an Englishman and translated into Latin by a Dutchman. The book is very pleasant and curious, but very delicate and mystical. You will receive it in the first package or by the first way that I may find. . . . The author does not lack spirit, you will see in it strange and ravishing thoughts. There is yet scarcely a book of this sort. If it be permitted to the wise to write thus freely one would learn much of novelty, there was never a Gazette worth it. The subtlety of the human mind can show itself in this way.

Again in a letter to Spon on April 16, 1645, he writes:

They make a great deal of the book entitled "Religio Medici." Its author has ésprit. There are a good many things in the book. He is an agreeable melancholic in his thoughts, but he, in my judgment, searches a master in religion like many others, and perhaps in the end he will not find one.

It is rather surprising to find Patin writing to Spon (July 26, 1650) in terms implying admiration of the eccentric spagyrite and Rosicrucian, Sir Kenelm Digby (1603–1665), the inventor of the famous "sympathetic powder," because if ever there was a believer in occultism, it was that doughty English knight. Be that as it may, Patin writes:

M. le chevalier K. Digby, an English gentleman, a very zealous catholic, learned and curious, has written while journeying, as he has done much for twenty years, chiefly in Italy, a Treatise on the Immortality of the Soul, in English printed today at Paris. It is this same Knight who has written also in English against the author of the book entitled Religio Medici. I ardently wish that that which he wrote of it was also put in Latin, seeing that I have a high opinion of these two minds (ésprits).

Of another Englishman Patin writes to Belin, *fils* (October 28, 1659): "Bacon was a chancellor of England who died in the year 1626, who was a great personage, of an elevated and curious mind. All that which he has done (written) is good."

When Thomas Hobbes, the English philosopher who wrote "Leviathan," was ill in Paris in 1651, Patin attended him. He writes Falconet (September 22, 1651) that Hobbes suffered from an attack of vomiting, with a greatly distended abdomen, and much pain. Patin, of course, proposed to bleed him but Hobbes refused to allow him to do so, objecting on account of his age, which was sixty-four years.

The next day, having insinuated myself a little more into his good grace, he permitted me to bleed him, which gave him a great relief. He alleged to excuse himself that he did not think one could take so much bad blood from him at his age. After that we were comrades and great friends. I allowed him to drink all the small beer that he wished. At last after a little purgation he was in good condition. He thanked me very much, and said that he would send me something good from England. May he soon return there gay and joyous, without any further hope of recompense.

Patin hated bitterly the Jesuits and all other ecclesiastics who mingled in affairs of state. To the Jesuits he frequently referred as "that Spanish and loyolitic vermine" or "the black troop of disciples of Père Ignace," and the "carabins de Père Ignace." "The world has been in perpetual trouble since the monks put their nose in its affairs. The philosophic liberty of physicians prevents them from loving much this sort of men."[9]

In several places he terms the Jesuits "the executioners of Christianity." Writing to Spon (November 16, 1643): "These executioners follow *à la fin* every occupation imaginable, provided there is something to be gained by it."

Patin,[10] writing of a book by Isaac de la Peyrère in which the author argued for the existence of a race of men on earth before Adam, the pre-Adamites, says there are others who claim that the inhabitants of Australia and America are not descendants of Adam but belong to a totally different creation. "These are curious men, gazetteers of another world, very like our preachers, who often let themselves go, telling us marvels of a country where they have never been and to which they will never go."

[9] Letter to Belin, May 20, 1632.

[10] Letter to Spon, September 14, 1643.

Patin in a letter to Falconet (June 17, 1659) quoting the Greek philosopher who when dying consoled himself with the reflection that in the other world he would be with good men, philosophers, poets, and physicians, adds: "I am of the same mind. If I could meet Cicero, Virgil, Aristotle, Plato, Juvenal, Horace, Galen, Fernel, Simon, and Nicolas Pietre, R. Moreau and Riolan, I would not be in bad company. There will be that to console me. I believe that there are many good men in that country in recompence for this, where they are very rare."

FRIENDSHIP WITH NAUDÉ

One truly human friendship Patin had, with a most congenial soul, namely, Gabriel Naudé, the famous librarian of Cardinal Mazarin. Naudé was born at Paris in February, 1600. He and Patin were fellow medical students in 1622. He received the degree of Doctor of Medicine from the University of Padua in 1628, but does not seem to have ever practiced medicine, devoting himself entirely to books, first as librarian to President de Mesmes, then as librarian and secretary to Cardinal de

Bagny, at whose death he served Cardinal Barberini in the same capacity at Rome, and afterwards Richelieu. In 1643 he assumed charge of the wonderful collection which Mazarin was gathering together. This amounted at the latter's death to 45,000 volumes, and owed its great value largely to the judgment and erudition of Naudé. In 1623 Naudé had published the book by which he is probably best known today, "Apologie pour les grands hommes soupçonnez de magie," which was translated into English by J. Davies in 1657, under the title, "The History of Magic, by Way of Apology for All the Wise Men Who Have Been Unjustly Reputed Magicians, from the Creation to the Present Age." In 1627, while still librarian for President de Mesmes he published his "Avis pour dresser une bibliothèque," which went through a number of editions and was translated into English by John Evelyn, and published in 1661, with the title "Instructions Concerning Erecting of a Library."

Many amusing stories were told of Naudé by his contemporaries. He bought books in quantity by weight and measure, instead of by title or volume. Walking into a bookshop he would scan a pile of books, not

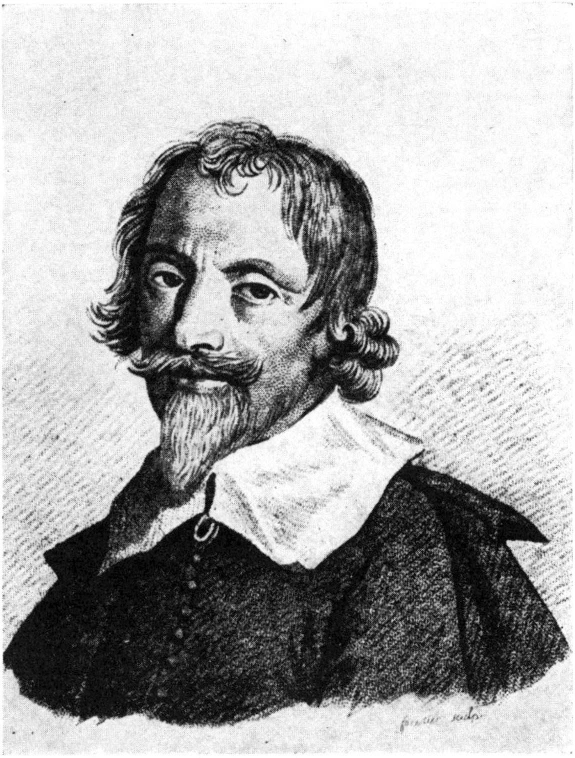

Gabriel Naudé
(1600–1653)

paying any attention to the individual volumes, and then offer the dealer so much per pound or foot for the lot. Taking them home he would sort them out, placing some in the Cardinal's library, buying some for his own which was very large, and then selling the duplicates. He was in the seventh heaven of happiness in his position with Mazarin. Although the great Cardinal was avaricious to the last degree, he would spend his ill-gotten gains like water for additions to his library. He sent Naudé all over France, and to Italy, Germany and England in quest of them. He is first mentioned by Patin in a letter to Belin, dated May 14, 1630, stating that he is sending him a small book which is the "Paranymph" for the year 1628," written by a very learned young man named M. Naudé." Its subject was after Patin's heart: *De antiquitate et dignitate scholae medicae Parisiensis panegyris; cum orationibus, encomiasticus ad* IX *iatrogonistas laurea medica donandos.*

Naudé figures frequently in Patin's correspondence. On August 27, 1648, he writes to Falconet a most amusing little skit about a projected trip which he, Gassendi and Naudé have planned for the following Sunday. The three are to go out to supper

DE
ANTIQVITATE
ET DIGNITATE
SCHOLÆ MEDICÆ
PARISIENSIS
PANEGYRIS,

CVM ORATIONIBVS ENCOMIASTICIS AD IX. Iatrogonistas laureâ Medicâ donandos.

Auctore GABR. NAVDÆO, Parif. Phil.

Diuitijs animosa suis.

LVTETIÆ PARISIORVM,
Apud IOANNEM MOREAV, viâ Iacobæâ, sub signo Globi Cælestis.
M. DC. XXVIII.
CVM PRIVILEGIO REGIS.

TITLE PAGE OF "DE ANTIQUITATE" BY GABRIEL NAUDÉ, 1628.

and to spend the night at Naudé's house at Gentilly:

There make a debauch, but God knows what debauch. M. Naudé drinks nothing but water, and has never liked wine. M. Gassendi is so delicate that he would not dare to drink it, and imagines that his body would burn up if he had drunk of it . . . for me, I can but throw sand on the writing of these two grand men; I drink very little, and nevertheless it will be a debauch, but philosophic and perhaps something more, for to be all three cured of night wolves (*loupgarou*) and delivered from the evil of scruples, which is the tyranny of consciences, we will go perhaps until very near the sanctuary. The past year I made this journey to Gentilly, alone with him tête-a-tête, there were no witnesses, also none were missed; we talked freely of everything, without anyone being scandalized by it.

On November 16, 1652, Patin writes to Belin, *fils*, that Naudé has gone to Sweden, where he had accepted the position of librarian to the eccentric Queen Christina, but his stay there was short, as in May, 1653, Patin writes that all the French whom the Queen had gathered about her, had been discharged from her service except Naudé, whom she wished to remain, which he refused to do, preferring to leave with his fellow-countrymen. Naudé lived a short time afterwards; his death occurred at Abbeville in July, 1653, as he was returning to France at the bidding of Cardinal Mazarin who had returned to power.

The only criticism Patin writes of Naudé is contained in a letter to Spon (March 22, 1648) in which he says that Naudé had been to see him and had complained of the avarice of Mazarin in that he had paid him very little for the services that had been rendered him:

> I think it is the fear of dying before having amassed wealth to leave to his brothers and nephews of whom there are a great many. And by this example I see easily that the passions enter just as much as ever in the minds of philosophers. I am however very sorry for it seeing that he is an honest man and worthy of better treatment by such a master (as the Cardinal).

Naudé was a freethinker. In an undated letter to Falconet, written in 1662 or 1663, Patin expatiates at length on the opinions and character of his deceased friend. He thinks he had been inspired with indifference about religion during his residence of twelve years at Rome, also that his unbelief had been fostered by one of his teachers, a professor of rhetoric at the college of Navarre. Of his personal character he speaks most highly. He was prudent, wise, well regulated, with "a certain natural equity" and a good friend, "no swearer, mocker nor drunkard. He drank only water and I never heard him knowingly tell a falsehood. He hated hypocrites, those who had once deceived him, and liars." In one of his books he asserted that Jeanne d' Arc had not been burned but that an effigy of wood had been consumed instead. Patin refers to a number of authors who have written that she really did suffer at the stake, and adds:

> For myself I am very strongly for this girl who has been an excellent heroine. I believe that all the miracle was political and beautiful finesse painted with the sacred and holy name of religion; which leads the world by the nose . . . I have, moreover, heard it said that she was not burned but returned into her country, where she married and had children.

Of course such detractions arise concerning almost all the great figures of history, but the authenticity of Jeanne d' Arc's story has been established beyond question. Not to speak of her recent canonization by the Roman Catholic Church, the records of whose heroes and heroines do not always bear too close scrutiny, the investigations of historians have unearthed legal evidence and contemporary statements which amply confirm the historic narration of her murder in the market place at Rouen. As to the miraculous fictions about her mission they merely detract from the grand simplicity of her story.

Naudé was not a very gallant man. He said: "I could never bring myself to get married. The way is too thorny and difficult for a studious man."[11]

During the troubles of the Fronde, after the Court had left Paris the Parlement of Paris, after proscribing Mazarin, ordered that his library should be sold. Patin writes Falconet (January 30, and March 5, 1652) about the sale:

All Paris goes there as to a procession. I have so little leisure that I cannot go, joined to which the librarian, who had charge of it, is M. Naudé my friend of thirty-five years,who is so dear to me that I cannot bear to see this dissolution and destructon. . . . Sixteen thousand volumes have already gone, there remain but twenty-

[11] Naudeana et Patiniana, Amsterdam, 1703.

four thousand. . . . M. Naudé, who is very angry against the Parlement, has bought all the books on medicine for 3,500 livres.

The King finally intervened and stopped the sale by a letter to Fouquet, the procurer-general, in which he also ordered that the money obtained be refunded and the books restored, as much as possible. In his will Naudé bequeathed the books that he had bought from Mazarin's library back to the Cardinal and the latter bought the rest of the books in Naudé's collection, so that they all became part of the great Mazarin Library in which they still remain. Queen Christina and many others who had purchased books at the sale, followed Naudé's laudable example so that when, in 1660, the Cardinal died leaving an immense sum of money and his library to form the Collège de Quatre Nations, the greater part of the books that Naudé had collected for him were again brought together.

CHAPTER V

Patin in Relation to His Students and His Sons

The younger son of his friend Belin[1] came to Paris to study medicine and Patin welcomed him to his house where, for a time, he came frequently. Then he remained away. Patin examined him at every visit. After a lengthy absence the examination was not satisfactory and Patin advised his father to take him back to Troyes. One can easily divine that the young man's visits to Patin were not an unmixed pleasure, for Patin thought he was indulging in debauchery. Patin's letters about him to his father are very kindly worded. In 1646 young Belin ran away from Paris and joined the army, owing Patin money and what was worse not having returned some books which Patin had lent him. Sometime afterwards young Belin wrote to Patin telling

[1] This was not the Belin, *fils*, with whom Patin corresponded. His letters were addressed to Claude Belin II; the lad who studied at Paris was yet another Claude, according to Triaire, who was registered as a physician at Troyes in 1654.

him with whom he had left his books, thereby reconciling himself to him, and later wrote again asking Patin to intercede with his father for him.

Patin wrote to Belin, *fils*, on October 17, 1642, an interesting letter of advice as to the reading the young physician should pursue:

Read only Hippocrates, Galen, Aristotle, Fernel, Hollier, Duret, Sylvius, Riolan, Tagault, Joubert, and very little of others, *in quibus Hofmannus ipse dux regit examen.* I am having printed here another book by him, of which I will make you a present in about a month as the author himself has sent it to me. Read the good theses of our school. Look at those which you have of them, to the end that I may send you the best if you have them not. While you have a little leisure, read all that Thomas Erastus has written and especially "De occultis pharmacorum estatibus," and his four volumes "Adversus novam medicinam Paracelsi." Read also every day the "Aphorisms," the "Prognostics," the "Prorrhetics," the "Epidemics or the Coaques" of Hippocrates. On the "Aphorisms," take of all but three commentators; to wit, Heurnius, Hollier, and Galen.

Again he tells young Belin, October 24, 1646:

Read every day some good book, and learn by heart, if you do not know them already all the

"Aphorisms" of Hippocrates . . . Do not let any day pass without studying at least eight hours. Read carefully the "Pathology" of Fernel and the first four books of his "General Method"; add to it the practice of J. Hollier, with the "Enarrations" of M. Duret, and the "Aphorisms" of Galen, of Hollier, and of Heurnius. The best surgeries[2] are those of J. Tagault and of Gourmelin.

There are three treatises by Galen which you should choose and frequently read something in them, to wit: "De locis affectis; de morborum et symptomatorum causis et differentiis," and his books on the "Method." You will do well to add that which he wrote by way of commentaries on the "Epidemics" of Hippocrates. If you desire another pharmacy than the "Method" of Fernel, read Renodaeus but do not let yourself be carried away in the current of so many promises as do the antidotaries who are destitute of experience. Nevertheless it is necessary to know something of compositions for

[2] It will be noticed that throughout his correspondence Patin never recommends the surgery of Paré, except when he himself added anonymously a treatise on fevers to a posthumous edition of Paré's works, but even then he does not refer to any excellence on the part of Paré's own books. Gourmelin was the bitter enemy of Paré and it was in reply to his attacks that Paré wrote his "Apology and Journeys in Divers Places," 1575.

fear that the apothecaries *artis nostrae scandala et approbria,* can take the bar over you . . . Do not lose your time reading many of the moderns who only make books of our art from lack of practice, and from having too much leisure. Above all flee books on chemistry, *in quorum lectione oleum et perdes.*

It should be noted that, in a certain sense, Patin was not a reactionary. He was an upholder of the Old Greek medicine, that of Hippocrates and Galen, against the pseudo-Greek medicine of the so-called Arabian school. For many centuries the Arabians had captured the preeminence in medical teaching and belief. The works of Avicenna, Avenzoar, Rhazes, and their fellows were the guides on which the medical profession of Europe founded their faith until well into the sixteenth century, and the Arabic traditions died hard, lingering into the seventeenth century. The new school comprised those who had taken up the new remedies introduced by Basil Valentine, Paracelsus, Van Helmont, de Mayerne, and many others. As these chemists compounded many formulae and believed implicitly in the efficacy of their various preparations against diseases, Patin could not see any good in their teachings. He only saw in them a new set of therapeutists who, like the Arabs, disregarded the teachings of the Greeks, as to the supreme importance of observation and diagnosis, and the *vix medicatrix natura*, in their desire to invent new remedies, and panacea. Other wiser but less prejudiced physicians than Patin, felt as he did that the salvation of medical practice lay in a return to the Greek tradition. Two men especially did much to promote this end. René Chartier, to whom Guy manifested such bitter enmity, published the works of Hippocrates and Galen in Greek and Latin with annotations, and Foesius published his magnificent Hippocrates in Latin, thus placing the works of the great master within reach of the many physicians who knew Latin but not Greek. There was a great division in Patin's time between the iatromathematical school, represented by Borelli and Sanctorius, and the iatrochemical school whose foremost representatives were Van Helmont, Franciscus de le Boë, or Sylvius, and Willis of England. The former held that all bodily actions and functions could be explained by the laws of physics. The iatrochemists held they were due to chemical activities in the organs and tissues. Patin's inclinations were evidently with the iatromathematicians, though he shows but little interest in the many great advances in anatomy which were made during his lifetime. He mentions the writings of men like Steno, Sanctorius, de le Boë, but chiefly praises or dispraises them for their typography or binding. He lauds highly those authors who adhere to the Hippocratic tradition and condemns virulently those who show any tendency to use the much detested "chemical" remedies, such as antimony. I have referred elsewhere to his views about Van Helmont. Harvey's book, the greatest contribution to medical science of his age, or for that matter any other age, the "De motu cordis" published in 1628, is only referred to in connection with the publication of books attacking his demonstration of the circulation of the blood by Patin's friend, Riolan, or by Primerose of Bordeaux.

Another young medical student for whom Patin acted as mentor at Paris was Noël Falconet, the son of Patin's correspondent, André Falconet. Their family contained many distinguished physicians. Charles Falconet was physician to Marguerite de Valois, the first wife of Henri IV. His son André, Guy's correspondent, was born in

1612, and died in 1691. He practiced medicine at Lyons. When his son Noël came to Paris to pursue his studies Patin manifested the same fatherly interest in him that he had shown in young Belin. Young Falconet came to Paris in 1658. When Falconet wrote to Patin that he intended to send him there the latter replied (September 24, 1658), advising him to keep him at home rather than send him to Paris:

Here the youth are marvelously debauched. You would make him a physician? He could study his philosophy at Lyons and later you could send him here for one or two years to study medicine. If your son remains near you, you will be more his master, his health will fortify itself, and he will be more capable of believing me in a year, if I am yet here. When he shall have studied here sometime, it will be necessary to make him pass doctor (get his degree) in a short time, and afterwards retire him near you, when he will follow you to your patients, and learn more in three months than in four years at Montpellier, where I hear that the young men are very debauched. I have many examples of it but take little interest in them. Being at Lyons near you, he can render you a good account of his leisure and at his ease and to his great profit he will read Hippocrates, Galen, Fernel, and Duret . . . If you retain your son at Lyons to study his philosophy, try to make him study Greek as well so that he will know his grammar, the New Testament, Lucian, Galen, and Aristotle. In two years he will be more robust and better able to stand his first winter at Paris, which is extraordinarily severe for newcomers and to the young, and even then he should be sent here in the month of August so that he may pass the autumn here and become accustomed (acclimated) before the winter comes.

Falconet did not take this sage advice but sent his son to Paris in the autumn of 1658. Falconet asked Patin to take him to live with him as a house-pupil. Patin writes (October 29, 1658):

I have never wished to take anyone *en pension,* although I have been asked to many times, but I can refuse you nothing. You talk to me of the price of board and lodging. I do not know what it is, I demand nothing of you. Tell me only if you wish him to study philosophy and what wine you wish that he should drink. For the rest he shall be nourished in our ordinary fashion, which will suffice a student.

Patin writing to Falconet (January 3, 1659) gives a pleasant picture of his home life and of the hospitality with which he treated his son. He tells him how the boy has enjoyed seeing the beautiful churches of Paris, and of some theological questions which they had discussed together, and how Noël goes frequently to see his son, Charles, at his house in the rue Saint-Antoine, "where he always sees something beautiful." Charles, being a numismatist, had many beautiful pictures and medals.

Often after supper warming ourselves about the fire, I talk to him of the great events of our history, of the deaths of the three kings, Henri II, Henri III, and Henri IV, of the deaths of the two Guises at Blois in 1588, of the Maréchal de Biron, of the Marquis d'Ancre, which I make him read near me in our historians. He says that Jacques Clément and Ravaillac, who killed Henri III and Henri IV (who I tell him were very good kings) were wicked rascals . . . He has a great wish to go there (to Cormeilles) at Easter with my wife, and see all our trees in blossom. We have there five hundred little pear trees without counting the prunes, peaches, apricots, mulberries, and fig trees, and will return from there to Saint-Jean where he will see two hundred cherry trees charged with ripe cherries. For three years I have had a great wish to take you there, but you have (when here) too much business; he will view them in your place. Our house is near the mountain on which we have a windmill from the top of which one sees the great spire of our church at Beauvais. We will show him that and teach him the topography of all the environs and suburbs of Paris.

When Chereau sought Patin's country house at Cormeilles he found only the cellars remaining, a new mansion having been built. There still existed vestiges of the windmill, and many cherry trees flourished on the grounds.

Guy's second and favorite son, Charles, "mon Carolus," was evidently a great friend of the young student. Patin writes Falconet somewhat later in the same month that Charles has promised to take Noël on the anxiously desired country trip at Easter.

In August, 1659, Guy tells of taking him walking and showing him the Latin motto on the great clock of the Palais de Justice, advising him to copy it as a good sentiment. Then they went to Cormeilles together, and on their return Patin took him to see the execution "of a thief who was broken on the wheel. They gave us a chamber from the window of which he saw all the ceremony of this mystery of destroying men for their crimes." This was done to inculcate a moral lesson, as Patin adds: "It was not without expatiating to him on the unhappiness of the wicked who resolve to steal and kill to have money for debauchery and gambling." Robert Patin was attending the wife of one of Mazarin's household who was ill at Vincennes, and he took his mother and young Noël Falconet in the carrosse with him when he went there one day in order to show them the chateau. Patin (October 6, 1659) telling the father about this little excursion, adds, "he promises marvels, God give him grace to do well."

Patin (April 6, 1660) writes Falconet:

Since you do not wish your son to go to Lyons for his vacation I am well content. He will eat of our good cherries and mulberries at Cormeilles, afterwards he will return here to learn the "Compendium" of Riolan, the father, and the "Enchiridium" of Riolan, the son. After that the winter will come, our public acts (demonstrations) and frequent dissertations will occupy him; you know these are the fundamentals of our profession. Finally he will study the pathology and general method of Fernel, with the "Aphorisms" of Hippocrates and the "Commentaries" of Hollier. I will make him write on paper the good things and practices. I will also take him to see patients where he will learn the *modus agendi*. All this can be done in thirteen or fourteen months and afterwards he can return to Lyons to see you and report to you on his studies.

Possibly young Falconet was aware of Patin's weakness and flattered him somewhat because Guy writes to his father (July 2, 1660):

Noël Falconet acquires every day some degree of wisdom, and will answer well. He greatly loves to be near me and hear me talk. Day before yesterday after dinner, as we were talking together, there came an honest man, with whom I talked about a half-hour, and then took him into my office to give him a prescription. This man, an officer of the king's, looked at him much and when we were alone he said, "that young man there listens to you attentively and wishes to learn. Ah! but if I was in his place I would profit by your presence."

Patin adopted the usual method of instruction, making his pupil learn from books and notes. He writes (August 10, 1660) that he is going to make Noël "learn by heart the first chapters of the 'Compendium' of M. Riolan, the father, and afterwards his commentaries on the physiology of Fernel, with the 'Enchiridium' of the son. It is the way I taught my two sons, and it succeeded there very well."

Apparently young Falconet only stayed temporarily at Patin's house because Guy writes his father (September 21, 1660):

Noël Falconet studies and often asks me good questions. I lent him some books to study but he wished to have his own, so I took him to the rue Saint-Jacques[3] and bought for him in his presence the works of Riolan, the father, in two volumes in octavo, and the "Enchiridium anatomicum et pathologicum" of the son. I have also promised him a "Perdulcis," and have lent him a Fernel in folio which he likes. He wishes

[3] The rue Saint-Jacques was the great bookshop center of Paris at that time. Patin's correspondence, as would be expected, is full of references to this famous thoroughfare. He writes to Belin on August 17, 1652 of a book which Belin had demanded, "I will have it tomorrow if it is to be found in the rue Saint-Jacques," and he writes jokingly to Charles Spon on November 16, 1645, that if the Pope ever comes to Paris he will go to see his entry and "await him in the rue Saint-Jacques in a booksellers, reading some book." In this connection we also find Patin applying the term Latin to that part of Paris lying on the left bank of the Seine which is still known as the Latin quarter. In a letter to Spon (May 24, 1650) he says: "I went yesterday *au pays* Latin, where the University is, to a consultation to which I had been called by one of my colleagues for the son of a councilor of Rouen. I went by way of the rue Saint-Jacques. All our booksellers are marvelously dry and ruined."

also the "Anthropographia" of M. Riolan, and Hollier in "Aphorismos Hippocrates, quia conciliavit doctrinam veterum cum nostra methodo Parisieni," which is better than that of the Italians.

PATIN'S DOMESTIC CIRCLE

On October 10, 1628, Patin married Jeanne de Jeanson, the daughter of a rich wine merchant of Paris, whose mother was a daughter of the celebrated Miron, the provost of the merchants of Paris. Ten children were born of the union, four of whom attained adult age, namely, Robert, the physician; Charles, the physician and antiquary; Pierre, of whom we only know that he became a Master of Arts in 1649, and that he signed the certificate of decease of his father in 1672, and François, who became a soldier and was killed in a duel by one of his comrades at Plessis-Bouchard, October 9, 1658. He was buried in the church at Cormeilles the next day. Chereau[4] was shown by the curé at Cormeilles-en-Parisis an old parochial register containing the following entry:

Ce mesme jour, 10 Octobre, 1658, François agé d'environ dix-neuf ans, fils d'honorable

[4] *Union Médicale*, 1864, 2d series, xxiii, 401, 449.

homme Mr. Guy Patin, docteur régent en la Faculté de médecine de Paris, a esté inhumé en la chapelle, Nostre Dame: lequel François Patin a esté tué le jour précédent, par un sien camarade de guerre, entre Francomille et le Plessis-Bouchard.

As. there is no reference to the career or the loss of this son in Patin's letters, it may be presumed that there was an estrangement between the father and son.

To judge by the frequent references to his children in the Letters, Patin was a devoted father. He writes to Charles Spon (March 24, 1648): "I love children. I have six of them and it seems to me that I have not yet enough. I would be very glad to have another little girl. We have but one, who is so sweet and so agreeable that we love her nearly as much as our five boys."

Guy writes to Spon (May 25, 1648) with curious candor about his wife's relatives:

For eight whole days I have been detained near my mother-in-law, who has been very ill with a pleurisy of which she, Dieu merci, was quit, by means of four bleedings which she has borne very well, in as much as she is nearly eighty years old. The good man is scarcely less, and they are on the eve of leaving me for my part an inheritance of 20,000 crowns, *et vir sapiens non abhorrebit.*

Patin's father-in-law showed no inclination to hasten the fulfilment of his hopes. Two years later (February 4, 1650) Patin writes Spon:

My father-in-law has again obtained some respite from the park (cemetery). In this last attack he was bled eight times from the arms, and each time I made them take nine ounces from him, although he is eighty years old. He is a fat and full-blooded man. He had an inflammation of the lungs with delirium, and, in addition, stone in the kidneys and bladder. After the bleeding I had him well purged four times with senna and syrup of pale roses, by which he has been so marvelously relieved that it is miraculous, and he seems rejuvenated. Many people would not have believed it and would believe rather some fable of a julep cordial. He shows me much contentment but although he is very rich he gives no more than a statue. Old age and avarice are always in good intelligence with one another. Such men resemble pigs which leave all in dying, but are only good for anything after they are dead because they are good for nothing during their life. It is necessary to have patience, I will not neglect to take good care of him. God has given me the means to do without the wealth of others, and live content till now without ever thinking evil.

Patin's mother-in-law died on July 8, 1650, and he wrote to Spon on July 26, 1650, and again on August 8, 1650, describing her last illness, an apoplexy, and rendering her a somewhat piquant last tribute. She was eighty-two years old. Patin was at Paris but hastened to her country place at Cormeilles where she was taken ill.

I found the good woman in extremity . . . She had been bled and cupped in awaiting my coming by the surgeon of the place, in such sort that there remained nothing for me to prescribe . . . Finally she died in the evening and was buried in the church there the next day with much ceremony, very useless and superfluous . . . We brought back the good man her husband the next day, who is more decrepit than she was although several years younger . . . There is hope that after his death we will have a great inheritance . . . She was an excellent woman in the care of her household and in the pains which she took with it . . . I can not give myself the pain of weeping much for her seeing she was too old and too often ill . . . Do not weep much for the death of my mother-in-law, she was not worth it. She was a good woman, very rich and avaricious, who feared nothing so much as death which nevertheless seized her quite suddenly at the end, at her beautiful country house at Cormeilles. She has gone before where we will go after. Let us try at least to go there with tranquillity and (better) reputation, and that our children may be thankful to us as good fathers, in meriting from them veritable gratitude.

Patin only refers to his wife in a very casual way throughout the correspondence. He speaks once of her pride in their good fortune as we have seen, but she seems not to have entered much into his thoughts or affairs. He hints at her rather disparagingly in a letter to Spon (October 5, 1657). The latter's wife had visited Patin at Paris and the latter writes:

Mon Dieu, but she is a worthy woman. Ah! but you are fortunate to have one so good, so perfect, and of such good humor. Mine has many very good qualities, but she is sometimes cross and cruel to valets and maids, which are characteristics I hold for nought, but she has them *Jure gentilitio*. Her deceased mother who lived eighty-four years was of the same humor. You have been more fortunate than others. Is it that God mixes in your affairs?

In a letter to Falconet (June 3, 1661) Patin makes the following ungallant remarks: "The late M. de Villeroi, grand secretary of state, who had a bad wife (he was not alone in that and the race is not extinct) said that in Latin woman was *mulier*, that is to say mule *hier*, mule *demain*, mule *toujours*."

ROBERT PATIN

As already stated, the Patins had four children who attained adult age. Robert, born in 1629, is frequently mentioned in the course of his father's correspondence. Some of Guy's letters are written in his hand, he evidently having acted as his father's secretary. Patin wrote to Spon in May, 1648, telling him of his joy that Robert had received his degree of Bachelor of Medicine at the age of nineteen, the youngest of his class. They quarreled on occasions and there was a serious breach between them at the end of Guy's life. In a letter to Spon in 1649, Guy wrote that Robert could do very well if he wished, but that he did not like to study and was volatile and flighty. He married Catherine Barré in 1660. Writing to Belin, *fils*, June 2, 1660, he says that two days before, he had married his eldest son to a beautiful girl, who comes of honest people, to whom he had been the physician for twenty-five years. "She is beautiful, she is rich."

Patin gave up his chair of *Professeur du roi* to Robert in 1667. He wrote to Falconet (August 12, 1667):

Yesterday my eldest son, Robert Patin, took possession of the charge of *professeur royal,* for which I had obtained for him the succession. It has come with a good augury, because he celebrated by his harangue his natal day, having been born the eleventh day of August, 1629. I pray God that he may enjoy it a long time. I have raised my children with great care and great expense. I hope they will reap agreeable fruits from it.

Robert died of phthisis on June 1, 1670. Chereau[5] gives the following entry from the register of the church at Cormeilles:

Le deuxieme jour de juin mil six cent soixante et dix a este inhumé dans l'église à la chapelle de la Vierge, Mr. Robert Patin, docteur en la Faculté de médecine de Paris, demeurant à la paroisse de Saint-Germain-de l'Auxerrois à Paris; en presence de Mr. Guy Patin, aussi docteur et professeur du roi, son père, et de Pierre Patin, son frère qui sont signé.

Although Charles was undoubtedly his favorite son, and Robert seems at times to

[5] *Union Médicale,* 1864, 2d series, xxiii, 401, 449.

have caused his father some vexation, nevertheless Patin was sincerely grieved when Robert died at the age of forty-one, but a few years after succeeding to Guy's professorial chair at the Collège Royal. In May, 1670, he refers on several occasions in his correspondence to Robert's illness, which seems to have made a rapid progress towards its end. He sent him, accompanied by his wife and his mother-in-law, out to his country place at Cormeilles in the hope that the change of air would help him. The bereaved father wrote Falconet (June 4, 1670):

At length, Monsieur, I am desolate, *O me miserum!* my eldest son died, the first of June. God wished to have his soul! he died a good Christian with great regret for his faults, *et cum maxima in Christum fiducia.* I pray God with a good heart that he will preserve you and those who belong to you. It is not necessary to go so soon, one dies soon enough . . . He died at Cormeilles, where he had been taken to have an air more pure than that at Paris. He was buried near his maternal grandmother and his brother François in the chapel of Notre Dame, near to the choir. *Requiescat in pace.* I am so broken down with sorrow at his death, and so fatigued by the journeys which his illness caused me to make, that I am capable of nothing. I pray you to witness my sorrow to M. Spon to whom I have not written of this misfortune because I am so much afflicted, and from whom I do not even ask consolation. It is necessary that I weep all my life for a son so learned . . . He leaves three boys and a little girl, of whom the eldest is nine years, and from whom I hope for some consolation, because he has much ésprit, learns well, and is very gentle. We will do that which pleases God, who holds in his hand the good and bad fortune of men.

In 1669, Robert according to Sue had gotten his father's signature to a document which enabled his wife to interfere in the disposition (*affaires*) of Patin's estate after his death, so that it was necessary to sell Guy's library of upwards of 10,000 volumes after his death, in order to satisfy her claims. The old man wrote to Falconet in July, 1671, a few months before his death, "that the diversity of the studies of his son Charles consoled him in some sort for his absence, but that the maliciousness of Robert confounds him." "This ingrate has deceived me wickedly, even while dying. I would never have thought that of an older son in whom I had trusted entirely."

CHARLES PATIN

Charles Patin was born on February 23, 1633, studied law and became an advocate at Paris in 1648, but in 1654 gave up his legal career and took up that of medicine. Patin tells Belin[6] that at the age of fourteen years he has been examined publicly in Latin and Greek philosophy, before a large audience and got his degree of Master of Arts. "I am going to put him back at his humanities for another year and then make him study law, so that some day he can defend me if the apothecaries undertake to attack me again." Writing to Garnier, a physician of Lyons, November 2, 1649, Patin says: "My Charles is studying law, but I would like it better if he would employ his time at medicine for which I find him much better suited. I talk to him of it often and he knows more of it than his elder brother; finally, I would prefer that he should be a physician rather than a law-maker, I would teach him many fine observations." In a letter to Spon in 1649, Guy says he is better poised and loves to study more than his brother Robert, and that he is very learned in "Greek philos-

[6] Letter, August 18, 1647.

ophy, geography and law." His portrait depicts a bright intelligent countenance of much physical charm. Writing to Spon (December 10, 1658) Patin tells him:

> It is very cold but we have wood to heat us, added to which it is warm in my study, and we study all the evening tête-à-tête until the hour for supper, and after that we talk around the fire of some agreeable matter, physics, history, or politics. Our Carolus always relates to us something curious. He loves ancient times and talks gaily of them to us, so much so that we often go to bed an hour later than we had resolved to.

He was apparently on the high road to success. He seems to have been a popular lecturer on anatomy, for Patin (December 16, 1659) writes to Falconet:

> My son, Charles, is teaching anatomy in our school on the cadaver of a woman. There is so great a number of auditors that besides the theater the court yard was filled. He begins well at twenty-six years, I hope he will finish better. He has many friends who love him. Through his studies he has acquired many and through his courtesy yet more.

On November 24, 1667, Guy wrote to Falconet describing with what éclat Charles had participated in a discussion on the relative merits of Homer and Virgil, and that Lamoignon, the President of the Parlement of Paris and one of the chief men in the city, had shown him marked favor, yet a few months later, in February, 1668, Charles had fled from France and was sentenced to the galleys in contumacy. Patin writes of it to Falconet (March 7, 1668) as follows:

I write lastly to you about the affair of my son in which I had expected that the knowledge of the truth and the succor of my good friends would have remedied it, but hope, according to the sentiment of Seneca, is the dream of a man who ages. Nevertheless, since it is a virtue, I would not abandon it whatever should arise, for it is permitted even to the most wretched to dream and to deceive themselves. Everybody pities him, no one accuses him, and with the exception of some publishers he is loved by everybody. Meanwhile he is absent and we are obliged to resign ourselves in spite of his stoicism. He had always hoped that the justice of the King would be extended to him but our enemies had too much credit. Meanwhile, to soothe our wound, they say, (1) that his process had been made in contumacy, as a man absent, who could not defend himself; (2) that it was by royal and special commission and without right of appeal which is extraordinary and shows more than ever the design they had to condemn him;

(3) that most of his judges had received *lettres de cachet* and the recommendation that it was necessary to make an example. But to what could this example serve? Is it that while the Hollanders and others print books of history, and chiefly of our country, of which the authors live in Paris, one can take from individuals the desire and curiosity to read them? (4) They allege it was a man of great standing who was our secret adversary who moved the wheels and intrigued against us, because they found among his books some volumes in defense of M. Fouquet, and of the enterprise of Gigeri.[7] Why do they not punish the authors of these books? Why do they not prevent their publication in Holland, or their importation into France? All these books, and others like them, have been sold at Paris by the booksellers at the Palais and in the rue Saint Jacques. It excites the desire to see these books that one would suppress and hide with so much rigor . . . They have named three books, to wit, one full of impiety, a Huguenot book entitled, "L'Anatomie de la Messe," by Pierre Dumoulin, minister of Charenton; as if the Inquisition was in France! It was sold for six sous. Paris is full of such books, and there is scarcely a library where one cannot find them,

[7] Patin evidently hints at Colbert in these remarks. It is well known with what animosity Colbert pursued all those who sought to uphold the cause of his predecessor.

even with the monks. There is liberty of conscience in France and the booksellers sell them every day. It is even permitted to a man to change his religion and become a Huguenot, if he wishes; and it will not be allowed a studious man to have a book of this sort; also he had only a single copy. The second was a book, which they said was contrary to the service of the King. It was the "Bouclier d'état," which is sold publicly at the Palais, and to which they are printing here two answers. The third is "L'histoire galante de la cour," which consists of little libels more worthy of contempt than anger. I think these three books are only a pretext, and that there is some secret enemy who is angry at my son, and the cause of our misfortune. I hope that God, time, and philosophy will deliver us and put us at rest, and in waiting, Lord God, give us patience. It is necessary in this world to be either the anvil or the hammer. I have never had great care, but here it is all of a sudden, when I am sixty-seven years old. It is necessary to bear patiently that for which there is no remedy. Finally God wills it thus.

Patin apparently did not think that Colbert was responsible for the persecution of his son, for when Colbert was ill a few years later, Patin writes Falconet (June 2, 1671):

For me I have a particular interest in his recovery, besides that he has often spoken well

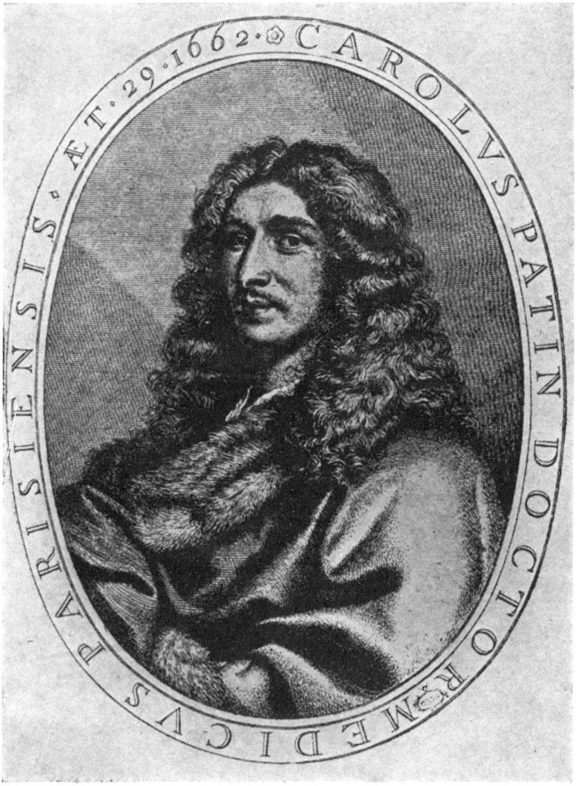

Charles Patin
(1633–1693)

of me, and that he has raised my salary as royal professor, it is that I expect from it the liberty of my son, Carolus, for although many persons have believed that it was he who had him persecuted, he has said several times, even of his own will (*même de son propre mouvement*), that it was not he. Thus we are reduced to knowing neither the accusation nor the accuser. But, as I have told you, I have good hope that this great minister will contribute to our happiness, in spite of the solicitations of our enemies.

On August 14, 1668, confirming a decree of the Châtelet previously issued March 25, 1668, Charles had been summoned before a special commission for trial without right of appeal. The only charge formulated against him was that certain prohibited books had been found in his possession: "L'anatomie de la messe"; the "Memoire" published by Fouquet in his defense; and Bussy-Rabutin's "Histoire galante de la cour," books which as his father says, were sold publicly by the booksellers of Paris. Guy Patin writes: "I think these three books are only a pretext and that there is some hidden party who is angry with my son and who is the cause of his misfortune." Bayle,[8] after quoting Guy Patin's explanations of his son's disgrace, says that they do

[8] Dictionnaire historique et critique.

not touch on the cause which was rumored about Paris as the true reason for his exile. It was said that Charles had been sent to Holland to buy up all the copies of a scandalous book, "Les amours du palais royal," and burn them at once, not sparing a single copy. He was given this commission by a "Grand Prince," who promised to recompense him. Charles was said to have purchased the books but instead of destroying them he was accused of bringing them into France where they would, of course, be in great demand. Pic conjectures, without giving any very valid reasons, that he may have become involved in a love affair with some lady upon whom the King had bestowed his affections. He bases his supposition on the facts that Colbert, the all powerful minister, had taken an active, though secret part in his conviction, the majority of the judges having received *lettres de cachet*, ordering them to find him guilty; that Charles Patin never attempted even while living in security in foreign parts, to justify himself, and that in 1681 he was offered a full pardon by Louis XIV. Charles refused the proffered amnesty, saying "of what pardon would they speak to me? I did not know my crime."

Pic recalls that Colbert had interested himself in the King's love affairs before, and that the trial of Charles Patin coincided in date with the advent to power over the King's affections of Madame de Montespan (1669), and that the pardon had been offered to him, without solicitation at the epoch of her displacement by Madame de Maintenon (1681). He thus accounts for the personal interest taken by Colbert and his royal master in the affair.

There does not seem much to support the idea that the exile of Charles Patin may have been due to a love affair. His wife followed him in his exile and apparently they lived with one another until parted by death, in perfect accord. There is another explanation for his persecution which seems more probable. In 1665, Denis de Sallo founded the *Journal des Savants.* Patin writes to Falconet (March 20, 1665):

I do not know if you have received a certain kind of gazette, which they call the *Journal des Savants,* in which an author who complained against a little article of my son, Charles, on the deal which was made here last year for the Swiss, is answered by him. I have sent you his answer, which is wise and modest. The new *Gazette* replied ignorantly and extravagantly, to which there had not lacked a strong and sharp response with good reasons, if they had not prayed Charles to suspend his reply, and menaced him with a *lettre de cachet*. The truth is that M. Colbert takes under his protection the authors of this journal, which is attributed to M. de Sallo, counselor in Parlement, to M., the Abbé de Bourze, to M. de Comberville, to M. Chapelain, etc., insomuch that Carolus is advised to delay his response, and even, by the advice of the premier president, who has also requested it (they say for a particular reason, to wit, that he does not stand well with M. Colbert since the process of M. Fouquet) . . . The republic of letters is for us, but M. Colbert is against, and if my son defends himself, they say they will send him to the Bastille. It would be better not to write.

This was not the only time that Charles Patin had been in trouble with the police for having in his possession contraband books. Pic's friend, M. Paul Delalain, discovered in the Bibliothèque Nationale the *dossier* of Charles Patin containing his sentence in 1668. Attached to it was the report of the arrest of both Charles and his father for an attempt to smuggle contraband books into Paris. They were bringing them into the city from Bourges, when their carriage was stopped and the two doctors apprehended and taken to the *douane*.

Among the books were ninety-two copies of Rabelais, the "Lettres provinciales," the *Journal des Savants*, "L'histoire des amours d'Henri IV," "Rome pleurante," "Le Roman comique de Scarron," and fifty copies of "L'histoire amoureuse des Gaules." The latter Guy Patin attempted to dispose of by throwing them down a latrine, but he was caught by the customs officers, and the books recovered by scavengers. There is no record of any punishment meted out for this offence beyond confiscation of the books.

In 1666, Guy and Charles Patin were arrested for having in their possession contraband books.

Again in 1667, the elder Patin was in trouble for the same cause. Fifty copies of the works of Hoffmann (Hoffmann's "Opera omnia") were found in his possession, and confiscated. "They were destined, not for presents, as he claims, but to be sold, according to his custom." After escaping from France, Charles Patin traveled and lived in England, Germany, Holland, Switzerland and Italy. He held several professional chairs at Padua, among them those of surgery and practice.

Patin was cheered by letters from Charles, showing that he had been well received in his wanderings, and was not greatly depressed by his banishment. Thus Patin writes to Falconet (September 13, 1668):

I have had good letters from Germany. By them I learn that my dear son, Charles, diverts himself there in traveling, and visiting worthy men. He has lately been at Frankfort, where our good friend, M. Scheffer, received him very well, also M. Lotichius, M. Horstius, and other men of letters. He writes me that he studies, and that he does not afflict himself too much at quitting his country. *Securus sine crimine vivit.* The Elector Palatine wished him well, and invited him to dinner twice a week, and asked him to all the amusements of the Court. He has even offered to write to the King on his behalf, but Charles is a Stoic, who says he does not wish to owe his return to anyone but the King. He says he is a wise Prince. They have persecuted him in his name, but that he will cause him to return when he wishes. If that does not happen, I will say with Cayas and others, *O ingrata patria, non habebis ossa mea!* I have more wish to see him than he has to return. My God, when shall it be?

Patin writes Falconet (April 26, 1669):

My Carolus has left Heidelberg and has gone to see the Duke of Wurtemberg, who has demanded his medical aid. He has already made another journey there, with which he was well content, as the Prince was also with him, sending him away with handsome presents, and charging him to return soon to see him. He writes me that if he loved money he would have the occasion to be satisfied, and that besides his profession in which they honor him much (you know that which is the honorarium of physicians and lawyers), these princes love greatly to play at tric-trac with him and they willingly lose. He says they are the honestest players and best men in the world.

Charles published a little book of travels[9] which contains nothing indicative of any great erudition on the part of the author, reading more like the jottings of an idle dilettante than a work written by a learned antiquary.

In 1682, Charles Patin published a volume of "The Lives and Pictures of the Professors at the University of Padua,"[10] including his own life and portrait as professor of surgery among them. This autobiographic sketch, however, is disappointing in that it throws no light on the reason for his exile. He relates with complacency

[9] Relations historique et curieuses de voyages en Allemagne, Angleterre, Hollande, Bohème, Suisse, par Charles Patin, Docteur en Médecin de la Faculté de Paris. Amsterdam, 1695.

[10] Lyceum Patavinum. Sive icones et vitae professori. Patavii, MDCLXXXII. *Publice Docentium.*

LYCEVM PATAVINVM,

Siue

ICONES ET VITÆ PROFESSORVM,

PATAVII, MDCLXXXII. PVBLICE DOCENTIVM.

PARS PRIOR,

Theologos, Philoſophos & Medicos complectens.

PER

CAROLVM PATINVM, EQ. D. M.

DOCTOREM MEDICVM PARISIENSEM,

Primarium Chirurgiæ Profeſſorem.

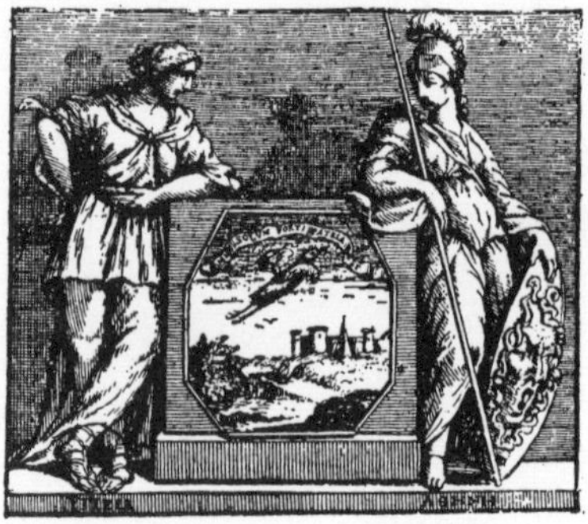

PATAVII, MDCLXXXII.

Typis Petri Mariæ Frambotti. *Superiorum permiſſu.*

Title Page of "Lyceum Patavinum" by Charles Patin, 1682

the many honors he has received since leaving his native land, and expresses the happiness which filled his life at the time he wrote. He refers with affectionate respect to his father.

Patin writes Falconet (June 19, 1663) of Charles Patin's marriage, speaking as though he were doubtful of its success:

> I have married my son, Carolus, aged thirty years, to the daughter of my colleague, M. P. Mommets. Her name is Madelon, and she is nineteen years less four months old. A beautiful girl, well born and well brought up by a good father and a wise mother, *Utinam omnia fauste succedant.* It is a bargain of which I am doubtful as to the success; *uxori atque viro est fatalis.*

His wife and daughters were very learned and all published books on various subjects. Charles died at Padua on October 2, 1692.

CHAPTER VI

Opinions of Patin

THE PHARMACOPEIA OF PARIS

In a letter to Belin (January 18, 1633) Guy writes of the "Dispensatory" which the Parlement of Paris had ordered to be compiled by the Faculty in 1590. There was no official pharmacopeia or dispensatory (Guy elsewhere refers to it as an *antidotaire, guidon des apothicaires, etc.*) in France. The first one in Europe was that of Valerius Cordus published by order of the senate of Nuremberg in 1555, entitled "Dispensatorium pharmacorum omnium quae in usa potissimum sunt."[1] Patin says the French apothecaries used as textbooks the "Antidotaire" of Nicholas Praepositus of Salerno, first printed in 1471; and the "Dispensatorium Galenochemicum" of Renou (Renodaeus, 1608). The order says it was to be made by twelve members of the Faculty. The original members having died, those who replaced them allowed the work

[1] Triaire: Lettres de Guy Patin, 1630–1672, Paris, 1907.

to lapse, saying that such a publication would only serve to maintain the rascality of the Arabs to the profit of the apothecaries, and Guy[2] quotes the Pietres in support of this view adding that three grains of senna in a glass of water purge as well or more surely than a heap of arabesque compositions. He says the apothecaries do not like him for his practice but that the people are so tired of their barbaresque tyranny and bezoardesque cheating that it is easy to escape from their, the apothecaries', hands. According to Guy there is no better pharmacopeia than "'Le médecin charitable' reinseignant la manière de faire et préparer à la maison, avec facilité et peu de frais les remèdes propres à toutes les maladies selon l'advis du médecin ordinaire," written by Philibert or Philippe Guybert, which was immensely popular. Guy wrote a "traité de la conservation de la santé" which was added to the book in its seventeenth edition.

The Pharmacopeia of Paris was finally published in 1628, and entitled "Codex medicamentarius seu pharmacopoeia Parisiensi."

Years afterwards (July 20, 1656) we find him again writing Belin, that there is no

[2] Letter to Belin, 1643.

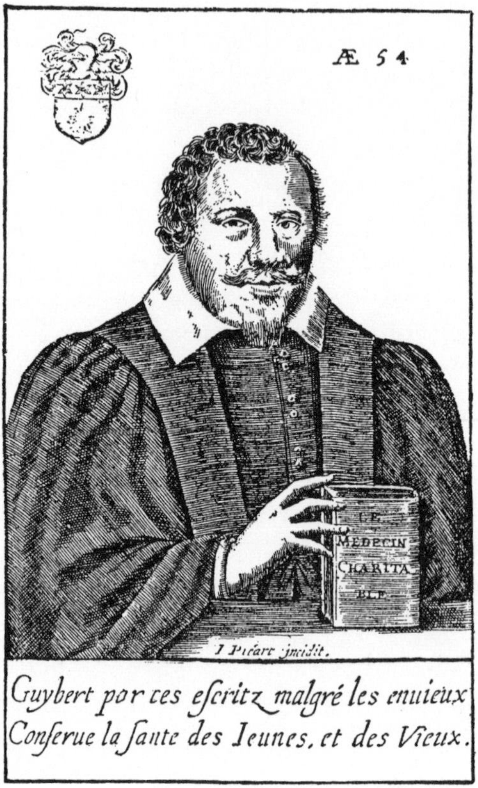
Æ. 54
LE MEDECIN CHARITABLE
I Picart incidit.
Guybert par ces escritz malgré les enuieux
Conserue la sante des Ieunes, et des Vieux.

FRONTISPIECE OF PHILIBERT GUYBERT'S "LE MÉDECIN CHARITABLE." PARIS: J. JOST. 1633.

better way to defeat the apothecaries than to introduce into families "Le médecin charitable" along with a syringe, bouillons and ptisans, made with senna and other emollient herbs.

PATIN AND THE BOOK TRADE

From the above it may be seen that Guy Patin though holding his head so high as a *docteur-régent*, was also a dealer in books to a very considerable extent. These commercial doings crop out with great frequency in his lectures. Whether he dealt in books to increase his income is doubtful. It would appear more probable that he was so intense a bibliophile that he could not refrain from handling them, whether in his library or in buying or selling. He seems to have enjoyed peculiar facilities for importing them and his activity in bringing foreign books into France was beneficent. He writes to Spon (September 17, 1649) about the efforts made by a syndicate of publishers to close the bookshops on the Pont Neuf. There were more than fifty of them, the privilege of opening them being sold by footmen of the King. Patin says they bought books stolen by children and servants and were a great annoyance to the regular trade.

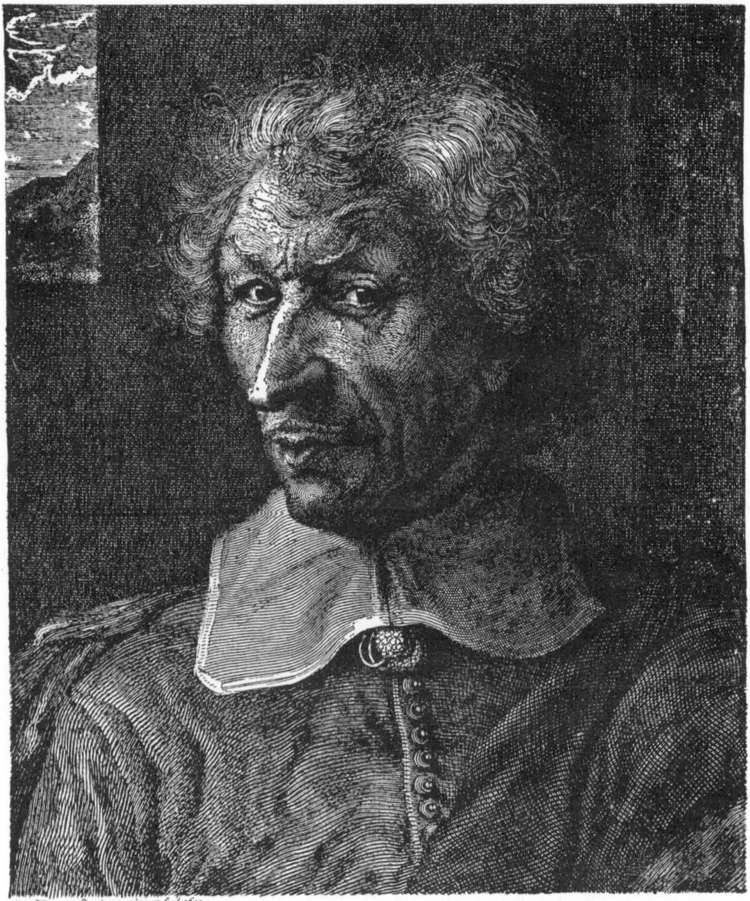

Me Guido Patin doctor medicus parisiensis medicus et professor Regius

(1602—1672)

In 1661, Patin besought the good offices of Falconet to secure the release of some books consigned to him, which had been seized by the customs officers at Lyons. A former student of Patin practiced medicine in Frankfort and when the great fairs were held in that city he used to buy books which he thought would interest his old teacher and send them to him. Patin was greatly concerned when he was informed that the package had been seized at the *douane*, on the complaint of the syndicate of the booksellers of Lyons. He writes that the only reason he can imagine for such action was that some of the books might be Huguenot, but he justifies the importation of such writings by the statements that Huguenot books are publicly brought into Paris and sold openly without any action against such trading on the part of the authorities.

When the elder Moreau died he left a very valuable collection of manuscripts and printed books to his son. The latter consulted Patin as to the best method of disposing of them. Four booksellers finally purchased the collection and arranged to dispose of them at public sale but Patin writes Charles Spon (February 16, 1657) that Fouquet, the celebrated procurer-general, stepped in and purchased all the medical books. Just why Fouquet should desire a medical library is not known.

Patin in a letter to Charles Spon (May 8, 1657) sounds a note about the publishers of Paris which resembles very much the complaints of the real lovers of good literature of the present time: "As to our publishers of Paris I can hope of nothing from them. They print nothing at their own expense but *novela utrisque sexus* (sex novels), I mean love stories or miserable books of the new piety, visions of the dreams of monks, of miracles and revelations, of cards of Saint Francis or girdles of Saint Margaret."

One of the chief publishers went into bankruptcy in February, 1658, and Patin writes to Charles Spon about it:

M. Cramoisy, who is king among the publishers of the rue Saint Jacques, has failed for more than three hundred thousand livres. This news surprises and marvelously astonishes me so much that I do not know who to trust any more among these dealers. I do not know how it could have happened, but I suspect that this man, who has printed so many books at the suggestion of the Jesuits, has warehouses

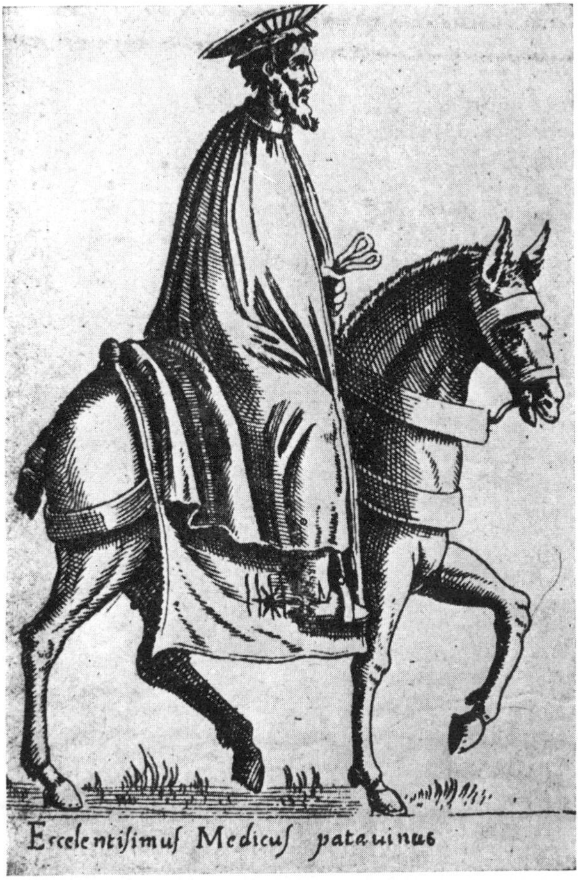

A PHYSICIAN MAKING HIS PROFESSIONAL CALLS IN PARIS IN THE SEVENTEENTH CENTURY

full of miserable merchandise that he cannot sell. This is a great misfortune for the book-trade, nevertheless I do not think that the carabins of Père Ignace will trouble themselves much about it, because these men, whatever money they may have care only for themselves, and practice craftily the old proverb, *primo mihi, secundo Michaud.* All the publishers of the rue Saint Jacques are greatly depressed but this stroke will mortify them yet more and diminish the little credit which they have.

There were two brothers Cramoisy. The younger fled but the elder who Patin says was a very honest man remained at Paris protected by powerful political and ecclesiastical influence.

Undoubtedly one of the "best sellers" of the time in France was the "Grand Cyrus" of Scudéry. Patin mentions in a letter to Charles Spon in January, 1654:

Sieur Scudéry who is an illustrious writer has finished his "Grand Cyrus, or Artamène,"[3] which is a very well received romance. He has written the "History of Alaric, King of the Goths," which they commence to print in a

[3] This was a mistake of Patin's as "Artamène ou le grand Cyrus" was written by Madeleine de Scudéry and "Alaric" by George de Scudéry. Patin had no use for the Scudérys, so was not particular as to detail.

folio, which will have many *tailles-douces*. Books such as these sell very well here to the courtiers, to the partisans and their wives, as well as the books of devotion, especially when it is some Jesuit or other monk of reputation who has written them.

On several occasions Patin refers with commendation to the books of Primerose, a physician of Scotch extraction, who practiced at Bordeaux. His two chief books were "Exercitationes et animadversiones in librum de motu cordis et circulatione sanguinis, adversus Guilielmum Harveum" (1630), and "De vulgi in medicina erroribus." Primerose was one of the most virulent and obstinate opponents of Harvey.

Gaspard, or Caspar Hoffmann of Nuremburg, another bitter opponent of Harvey's demonstration, was greatly admired by Patin, who published an edition of some of his works. Patin refers to him very frequently in terms of extravagant praise. When Harvey was traveling in Germany as physician to the Duke of Arundel he visited Hoffmann at Nuremburg for the purpose of demonstrating to him the correctness of his views. Vesling, whom Patin also mentions with much admiration was yet another opponent of Harvey, basing his objections on the different color of the blood in the arteries from that in the veins.

It is curious to witness such an obsession on the part of a man whose intellect was as keen as that of Patin. As a professor of anatomy, we know that he performed dissections, or at least lectured on bodies which had been dissected by his prosector for him. He was not however an original worker, probably contenting himself with reading anatomy to his students either from Galen or some contemporary whom he admired, such as Riolan, and not troubling himself to follow up on the body any of the wonderful anatomical discoveries of men like Harvey, Pecquet or Bartholin, to ascertain whether they were true or not.

PATIN'S HEALTH

Guy possessed good health. The physicians of his time made their professional visits on a mule or on horseback. Patin apparently did the latter; at least he writes to Spon (January 8, 1650) "that he had been out every day on horseback," and there is no mention in his correspondence of his ever having suffered any very serious illness during the seventy-two years of his life. The only indispositions he mentions are the following: Writing to Spon (March 10, 1648) he tells him that he has been ill with a bad cold that finally required him to take to his bed and undergo seven bloodlettings; in another letter (March 7, 1651) he tells him that some years before, after drinking polluted water, he had passed blood and pus in his urine but that it had soon cleared up.

He writes Belin (May 10, 1653) telling him that he had always been a very moderate drinker and ascribes to this the fact that he does not yet need glasses, "notwithstanding my age and my vigils."

Patin was consistent in applying his therapeutic views to himself when he fell ill. He tells Falconet (June, 1661):

> I had a bad toothache yesterday, which obliged me to have myself bled from the same side (as the pain). The pain stopped all at once, as by a kind of enchantment, and I slept all night. This morning the pain began a little again. I had the other arm bled and was cured right away. I am, thank God, without pain. I think that these two bleedings will serve to enable me to purge myself surely, which I shall do next week, if I have the leisure for it.

Although he followed the ancient Greek and Latin medical authorities with blind faith, it is interesting to note Patin's freedom from belief in some of the traditional remedies of his day.

Thus he writes to Belin, *fils* (October 18, 1631), at a time when a pestilential disease prevailed in Paris, that he does not believe that theriaca, mithridates, alkermes, hyacinth, bezoar, or the unicorn's horn are of any use, because he does not think they possess any of the occult properties attributed to them.[4]

[4] Theriaca, or treacle as his English contemporaries termed it, was regarded as a universal panacea against the bite of any venomous animal. It contained some sixty odd ingredients, among them bitumen, turpentine, saffron and vipers. It was invented by Andromachus, one of Nero's physicians, and was in great vogue even as late as the eighteenth century. Evelyn in 1646 records in his "Diary" that when in Venice he went to see its preparation, "the making an extraordinary ceremony whereof I had been curious to observe, for it is extremely pompous and worth seeing." In both France and Italy its manufacture was a long process attended with much ceremonial and many curious observances. The London Pharmacopeia for 1746 still retained it as official, as it also did mithridatum, a universal antidote supposed to have been invented by Mithridates, King of Pontus, and made of nearly as many ingredients as theriaca. Alkermes or kermes was, as its name would indicate, a product of Arabic pharmacy. It was made originally from cocoons which were found on a species of oak tree. It was especially

Patin writes to Spon (February 4, 1650):

The reputation of theriaca is without effect and without foundation, it comes only from the apothecaries who do all they can to persuade people to use compositions and would take from them if they could the knowledge and use of simple remedies which are more useful. If I were bitten by a venomous animal I would not trust in theriaca, nor in any cardiac, external or internal, of the shops. I would scarify the wound deeply, and apply to it powerful attractives, and only have myself bled for the pain, fever, or plethora. But by good fortune there are scarcely any venomous animals in France. In recompense we have Italian favorites, partisans, many charlatans, and much antimony.

---

famous in the form of the confection of alkermes. Hyacinth was not made of the plant of similar name, but from precious stones, especially amethysts. The confection of hyacinth contained many other ingredients, such as other stones, musk, myrrh, camphor and various herbs. Bezoar stones were concretions found in the gastrointestinal tracts of various animals, especially goats, llamas, and antelopes. Its use came from the Arabs and it was supposed to be a universal antidote for all poisons. Unicorn's horn was generally made from the tusks of elephants or narwhals, although supposed to be derived from the fabulous unicorn. Paré had fully exposed the uselessness of bezoar and unicorn's horn, though Patin never refers to his memorable treatise.

The pest of which Patin writes in the letter above quoted was the bubonic plague, as he says of it:

> There have been here since Easter a great quantity of malignant fevers, which have been as many hidden plagues, but one only names it the pest when one has seen buboes or charbons supervene, yet these diseases are not less contagious than the plague.

He complains that although there are two hospitals, Saint Louis and Saint Marçeau, in Paris, to which the plague-stricken were sent, there is no physician attached to either hospital to look after the patients. Patin says that he had seen more than sixty cases of plague himself, and that there was not a physician of the Faculté who could say that since the month of July he had not "seen, found or discovered nearly every day someone who was not a victim of it, because it has been very common here."

He tells Belin (October 2, 1631) of the heroic action of a physician named Malmedy who in the plague visitation in 1582 and 1583 voluntarily shut himself in the plague hospital without pay. Patin adds somewhat spitefully, that nevertheless he made a great deal of money in the hospital and lived to enjoy his gains for twenty years after, when he died of "pure old age."

Patin in a letter to Spon (January 8, 1650) makes a statement which goes far towards confirming the views of those who hold that syphilis was not imported into Europe from America, but that it existed in the Old World, but was regarded as a form of leprosy. During the medieval period and down to the beginning of the sixteenth century, leprosy was so prevalent throughout Europe that most communities of any size had leper hospitals to provide for its victims. At the present time leprosy is practically extinct in Europe, but syphilis is universally prevalent. Patin writes: "The late Simon Pietre, older brother of Nicolas Pietre, two incomparable men, said that before Charles VIII in France, the syphilitics were confounded with the lepers, of which today our hospitals are for the most part empty."

Patin refers again to this confusion in the diagnosis between syphilis and leprosy in writing to Spon (May 11, 1655):

> It is not long since I was shown a patient, an Auvergnat, who was suspected of leprosy, perhaps because his family had the reputation to have had it among them, because there was no

mark on his person. This made me think of some lepers here. In other times there was a hospital here dedicated to receive them in the Faubourg Saint-Denis, which is today occupied by the priests of the mission of Father Vincent (Saint Vincent de Paul). One sees them neither in Normandy, Picardy, nor Champagne, although in all these provinces there are leper hospitals which have been converted into pest hospitals, *Propterraritatem elephanticorum.* In other times they took syphilitics for lepers, *qui per inscitiam medicorum et saeculi barbariem, nec distinguebantum ab elephanticis, nec sanobantur.* Nevertheless there are still lepers in Provence, Languedoc, and Poitou. François Valleriola and Guilbert Ader assert it. Are there any in the Lyonnais? Have you seen any or recognized any as such? Have you in your city of Lyons a hospital for them? Have you seen them at Montpellier, or in any other places in Languedoc when you have been there?

Patin presents to Falconet (September 22, 1653) the historical and literary evidences of the antiquity of syphilis:

Bolduc, a Capuchin and Pineda, a Spanish Jesuit, have written that Job had syphilis. I am willing to believe that David and Solomon had it likewise. . . . In Hippocrates . . . and in Galen you can read about buboes, venereal ulcers, and gonorrhea. *Morbus campanus,* in

Horace, is syphilis. It is found in Catullus, Juvenal and Apulius, and they even say in Herodotus and Xenophon. M. Gassendi said to me that the leprosy of the Bible was syphilis. A libertine said that the serpent in Genesis was a young devil who gave Eve syphilis, and that was the original sin of the monks, so said M. de Malherbe.[5] At least it is certain that syphilis was well known in Europe before Charles VIII went to the conquest of the kingdom of Naples. . . . The late MM. Pietre, Riolan and Moreau were of the same opinion.

The introduction of the preparations of opium into practice undoubtedly led to considerable abuse of it at the hands of the incautious or unscrupulous. Its beneficent properties caused it to be hailed by many as the long sought panacea. The followers of Paracelsus were especially active in prescribing it often in harmfully large doses. It should be stated that the preparation which Paracelsus himself termed laudanum and recommended so highly, was not the tincture of opium to which we give that name today. The "laudanum" of Paracelsus was a gum or balsam called "ladanon," which was given in pill form. Patin, along with many of his contemporaries and those who

[5] Malherbe was the famous French grammarian and poet.

came later, confused the terms and thought the Paracelsan remedy was an opiate. Patin, with his usual combination of conservatism and prejudice, condemned laudanum and all other preparations of opium with the utmost vehemence. Thus Michel Potier, in his works published in 1645, having commended opium and some of the "chemical remedies," Patin attacks him bitterly in a letter to Spon (January 20, 1645):

I have heard said by M. Moreau, who was an Angevin like this Potier, that he was a great charlatan and a great rascal, who mixed in our profession, only showing himself on the stage to sell his wares better. He left the kingdom and made his way to Italy. Likewise he made himself in his book the Aristarch and censor of physicians. To hear him talk, it was he only that had knowledge and understanding. That which makes me suspect all he does is that he talks too often of his diaphoretic gold, of his opium or laudanum, and condemns too much the other remedies from which the people every day derive solace. His book is a continual censure of ordinary medical practice. Nevertheless there will always be fools who will admire him, and honest men will not gain any profit from him. This book will become ridiculous, or else it will render ridiculous all the profession of which we are part, you and I.

Patin does not condemn quinine, which had been introduced into France under the name of Jesuits' bark, as bitterly as he does antimony and opium, but, being a novelty, he cannot approve it. He writes to Spon (January 30, 1654) that he had dined with Gassendi and had met at his table a M. Montmor, *maître des requêtes*. This gentleman was a great collector of books and Patin was greatly delighted with him, especially when he intimated that he intended to employ him as his physician, but he adds that he has his doubts as to their according well together:

> M. Montmor has always loved chemistry and is not yet undeceived as regards antimony, and his wife also leans to these heresies; she is also for the Jesuits' powder, of which I have never seen any good effect in Paris.

On March 10, 1654, he writes Spon that the wife of de Gorris, one of his colleagues, had been found dead in her bed. She was sixty years old: "All winter she had suffered from a triple quartan fever, to cure which she had taken cinchona by which she thought she was cured. I think that this loyolitic powder (*poudre loyolitique*) shortened her days."

Imagine Patin thinking well of anything emanating from the Jesuits; could aught good come out of Nazareth? Patin writes to Falconet (December 30, 1653):

> This powder of cinchona has not any credit here. Fools run after it because it is sold at a very high price, but having proved ineffective it is mocked at now. I had treated a girl for a quartan fever so successfully that the access of fever was reduced to two hours only. Her mother, impatient, having heard the rumor made by this Jesuits' powder, purchased one dose for forty francs in which she had great hope because of the high price. The first access after this dose lasted seventeen hours, and was much more violent than any which she had had before. Today the mother has great fear of the fever of her daughter and much regret for her money.

The enlargement of the spleen, so frequently associated with malarial fevers, was recognized by Patin and his contemporaries, but the following extract from a letter to Falconet (September 21, 1661) will serve to illustrate the errors into which they fell because of the humoristic doctrine which dominated their views:

But apropos of quinquina, it performs no miracle here. When the body is well cleaned out by bleedings and purgatives, it is able by its (own) heat to absolve or absorb the remainder of the morbific matter, at least for that purpose it is only necessary to heat it. Even those in whom the fever has ceased are not entirely well, because it returns unless they are well purged. The obstinacy and duration of these quartan fevers comes from the bad, almost carcinomatous condition of the spleen, which occupies its very substance. I have never given cinchona. I have seen those who have trusted to it too much hydropic. I would not purge at the access of a quartan fever, but I purge often at the end of an access, with much success. Even in great fever, I sometimes make them swallow four great glasses of laxative ptisan, containing senna. That makes the bowels open well, carries off a portion of the conjoined cause, and prevents the annoyance of the great sweats, of which they complain so often. As to bleeding at the commencement of the access, I never do it. It would be both imprudent and temerarious to do so.

ORVIETAN

Orvietan was a quack remedy much in vogue in Patin's time.

Patin writes Falconet (January 6, 1654) of a curious episode in the Faculté de

Médecine in regard to it. He begins with a denunciation of de Gorris, a physician with a very large practice in Paris:

All his life he has been of the evil party of the chemists, the charlatans, the Gazetteer, the foreigners, the men with secrets against gout, epilepsy and quartan fever; a very unfortunate practitioner who has killed many with the experiments he would make. He knew truly much Greek and Latin, but applied his knowledge badly, and never had the courage to resist the temptation of gold for any rascality or corruption of his profession. In 1647, a merchant of Orvieto, to sell his drug better, addressed himself to a man of honor, then Dean of our Faculté, M. Perreau, to obtain through him by means of a good sum of money which he offered him, the approbation of the Faculté for his opiate. He refused it with much dignity. The charlatan then addressed himself to de Gorris, who received from him a considerable present and promised him to get some doctors to sign an approbation of his medicament which he sold on the Pont Neuf, which he caused to be done by a dozen of others who were hungry for money. These were the two Chartiers, Guénault, le Soubs, Rainssant, Beaurains, Pijart, du Clédat, des Fougerais, Renaudot, and Mauvilain. The Italian impostor, not content with such signatures, sought to have the approbation of the entire Faculté, and pressed the new Dean, whc was M. Pietre, my predecessor, to make him give it to him, in the hope which he had to make a better sale of his drug if he should obtain that which he desired. The new Dean learned from the charlatan's own mouth all that de Gorris had done for him, and when he had assembled the whole Faculté, and recited the affair against these twelve Messieurs, having acknowledged their weakness and bad action, they were expelled from the Faculté by a solemn decree. However they were reestablished on certain conditions, notably that of demanding pardon from the company in full assembly. No matter what they have been able to do since, the stain remains on them.

PATIN'S VIEWS ON INFANT FEEDING

Patin was a great believer in the nourishment of children by the maternal milk instead of on pap, which, as compounded in France at that time, was a mixture of wheat and flour, called *bouillie*. He thought that hand-fed babies were more subject to smallpox even in later life, and attributed his own exemption from that disease to the fact that he had been a breast-fed baby. He also thought that whooping-cough, which seems to have been as prevalent in France in his time as it is in our own, was predisposed to or aggravated by the artificial feeding of children. He describes whooping-cough in one of his own children, a little boy of three months, who had been taken out in very cold weather by his nurse. The illness lasted five weeks with paroxysms of cough lasting from a half-hour to three-quarters, during which time Guy thought him in danger of suffocation. "Two blood-lettings, enemata, good breast milk, abstinence from pap, and keeping warm are the great remedies."

Patin's particular objection to the use of pap was that it was "a coarse food which causes much stickiness and obstination in the stomach and abdomen, and which predisposes to illness of a putrid nature." He adds:

> I hold pap a bad food, as much because of the flour which is not often sufficiently good, as because of the milk of the cow, which is far from the goodness of that of the breasts, which is taken entirely fresh and new, hot and spirituous by the child, whereas that of the cow is extremely weak in comparison, joined to which it is a gross, viscous food which makes a stickiness in the stomach of the child, and much obstination in its belly.[6]

[6] Letter to Spon, January, 1644.

He also says that smallpox was unknown to the ancient Greeks, and that children got no pap in their time.

In Patin's time human milk was much esteemed not only as a diet for children but also under certain circumstances for adults. Patin (April 1, 1650) writes to Spon that d'Esmery,[7] the Superintendent of the Finances is very ill, and that Valot his physician has put him on a purely milk diet. "In the morning he drinks ass's milk, at midday cow's milk, in the evening goat's milk, and in between the milk of a woman." The Duke of Alva, one of the greatest and cruelest generals of his time, in his old age had two wet nurses by whom he was nourished, and Dr. John Caius, the famous English physician who founded Gonville and Caius College at Oxford, was, when senile, fed in the same manner. Shakespeare hints at this in the "Merry Wives of Windsor," when the Dr. Caius of the play has as his nurse, Dame Quickly.

Patin advocated the drinking of ass's milk, a measure much in vogue in his time, in cases of debility or prolonged conva-

[7] A creature of Mazarin's, his real name was Particelli. He was finally disgraced and replaced by Fouquet.

lescence. When Falconet's wife was recovering from a serious illness, Patin writes (April 8, 1664) urging him to make her drink it. He quotes instances to show Falconet that drinking ass's milk is conducive to longevity:

My mother-in-law, who died aged eighty-four years of an apoplexy, had drunk it for sixty years. The mother of M. du Laurens, the councilor, died last year, aged eighty-seven years, having used it ever since she was twenty-two years of age. Her sister-in-law, the widow of André du Laurens, the anatomist, had done the same and lived eighty-five years. It works marvels here, particularly in the spring and autumn, notably when taken with precaution. I only give it when the intestines are clean and prepared by good and gentle purgations.

VENESECTION IN INFANCY AND OLD AGE

It is hardly to be believed, but Patin asserts to Spon (August 17, 1658):

We also bleed very fortunately children of two or three months, without any inconvenience. I can show more than two hundred of them bled at this early age. There is not a woman in Paris who does not think well of bleeding and that her child should be bled in the fever of smallpox, scarlet fever (*rougeole*) or teething, or in convulsions, so much have they seen of it by experience when they had them.

Patin writes Falconet (January 19, 1663):

I bled another time an infant of three days for an erysipelas of the throat. He is still living, aged thirty-five years, a captain at Dunkirk, the son of Mademoiselle Choart.[8] I bled the son of M. Lambert de Thorigny the sixty-second day of his life, who is today ten years old. The application of great remedies at so tender an age demands much judgment.

The aged were also suitable subjects for profuse bleeding. Patin writes to Falconet (May 27, 1659):

Our good M. Baralis has been bled eleven times in six days, which has prevented suffocation . . . But he is in great danger of not being able to escape it. A continued fever, a bad lung besieged with an inflammation, eighty-four years, are all signs which leave me with a gloomy suspicion. Oh! but it is a pity. He knows well his Hippocrates and Galen, and practiced medicine as a man of honor all his life.

THE USE OF ANIMAL REMEDIES

It is odd that Patin neither recommends nor condemns a class of medicines much in

[8] It was quite customary at that time to designate a married woman as mademoiselle.

vogue in his time, namely those composed of animals or their secretions or excretions. Dr. Minivielle[9] gives the following list of those which the apothecary should keep in his shop, according to the "Pharmacopoeia" of Jean de Renou, published first in 1608 and again in 1637.

One uses many entire animals, such as cantharides, centipedes, worms, lizards, ants, vipers, scorpions, frogs, crayfish, leeches and many small birds. As to the parts (of animals) our physicians hold assuredly and truly that they are endowed with many and admirable virtues, among which parts we can put the skull or the head of a man dead but not yet buried; the bone which is in the heart of a deer, the brain of antelopes, swallows and hares; the teeth (tusks) of the boar and the elephant, the heart of the frog; the lung of the fox, the liver of the goat, the intestines of the wolf; the genitalia of the deer; the skin and the slough of the snake. Item: fat of man, of the pig, of the goose, of sheep, of the duck, the rabbit, the kid, the eel, and the snake; the marrow of the deer, the calf and the goat; human blood, the blood of the pigeon, and of the goat; all sorts of milk and that which is made from it, as butter and cheese; the horns of the deer, and antelope and the unicorn; the toe nails of the eland, the goat and

[9] La médecine au temps d'Henri IV.

the buffalo; the shells of oysters and the pearls from within them, and the scales of many fish. Finally, since the excrements of the said animals have also their particular virtues, it is not unfitting for the pharmacist to keep them in his shop, especially the dung of the goat, dog, swan, peacock, pigeon, muskrat, civet, and the hair of certain animals.

CHAPTER VII

Some of Patin's Contributions to Literature; Professor of Medicine

Patin edited a collection of discourses or harangues by Jean Passerat, professor of eloquence and Latin poetry in the Collège Royal, published in 1637, with a dedication to Charles Guillemeau, written by Patin. The edition of Fernel's "Pathology" (Fernelli Pathologiae), published at Paris in 1638, was prefaced by a dedication three pages long by Patin. Patin sometimes exhausts even his hyperboles in praise of Fernel. As a sample he writes to Falconet (March 29, 1656):

> I am ravished that you should so greatly love our Fernel. That man is one of my saints, with Galen and the late M. Pietre. I told Madame de Riaut, the mother of your beautiful nun, that I would hold it a greater glory to be descended from Fernel than to be King of Scotland, or related to the Emperor of Constantinople. Fernel was good, wise and learned . . . never any prince did so much good to the world as Fernel has done.

Fernel, physician to Henri II, was a truly great man. He was interested in astronomy, and in 1527, he tried to measure the earth's size by observing the height of the pole at Paris; then proceeding northward until its elevation was increased exactly one degree, and ascertaining the distance between the stations by the revolutions of the wheels of his carriage, he made it 24,480 Italian miles in circumference.

About the middle of the seventeenth century a physician of Paris, L. Martin, published a translation of "The Regimen Sanitatis Salernitanum" in burlesque verse, dedicated to Scarron. Some bibliographers have advanced the theory that the real translator was Patin, but Reveillé-Parise thinks there is no proof of the assertion. A later edition of this translation, published by Henault at Paris in 1651, is dedicated to Patin. Patin frequently refers to this translation, and in a letter to Spon (October 19, 1649) tells him that Martin, the translator, has shown him some of the pages of the proposed work and intends to dedicate it to him.

Writing to Charles Spon (December 3, 1649) concerning a dedicatory epistle which Spon was going to address to Patin as a preface to the works of Sennertus, Patin gives him a few hints as to what might be said about him, such as references to his books, his library, his patients, his good method of practice, his worthy inclination to do right in all things, to serve the public, to be neither charlatan nor chemist and to have good friends, both in France and in foreign countries.

Patin contributed considerably to various editions of the works of Jean Riolan, *fils*, adding tables and aiding in their correction for the press, and Triaire thinks it probable that he retouched his famous "Curieuses recherches sur les écoles en médecine de Paris et de Montpellier," published at Paris in 1651. Riolan states himself his indebtedness to Patin for his aid in his "Enchiridium anatomicum et pathologicum," 1648, which he dedicated to Patin.

Jean Riolan, the elder, who died in 1606, was Dean of the Faculté de Médecine from 1558 to 1559. His son, Jean Riolan, the younger (1577–1657), was professor of anatomy and botany at the Collège Royal, and physician to Marie de'Medici whose confidence he betrayed by spying on her actions for Richelieu. Although he denied the circulation of the blood and the existence of lacteal vessels and the lymphatic circulation, he made some advances, describing the fat appendices of the colon, naming the hepatic duct, and observing that the common bile-duct had but one membrane which served as a valve.

Jean Pecquet announced his discovery of the thoracic duct and receptaculum chyli in his book "Experimenta nova anatomica," published in 1651. Riolan, of course, combated his views, and Patin writes to Belin, *fils* on October 8, 1653: "There is an entirely new book by the goodman, M. Riolan, 'Adversus Pecquetum et Pecquetianos,' which is much approved and well received. All those who have read it wish well to M. Riolan, and mock the others, who are treated in a strange fashion."

Elsewhere Patin writes to Spon (March 26, 1655) and shows his pronounced leaning towards empiricism as contrasted with scientific research. He says:

For the new opinion of Pecquet, I do not yet make much of it, inasmuch as I can see no certain proof of it nor grand utility or information, *ad bene medendum.* He who discovered for us senna, cassia, and syrup of pale roses, has given us much more pleasure and has insulted no one, as these others have done M. Riolan

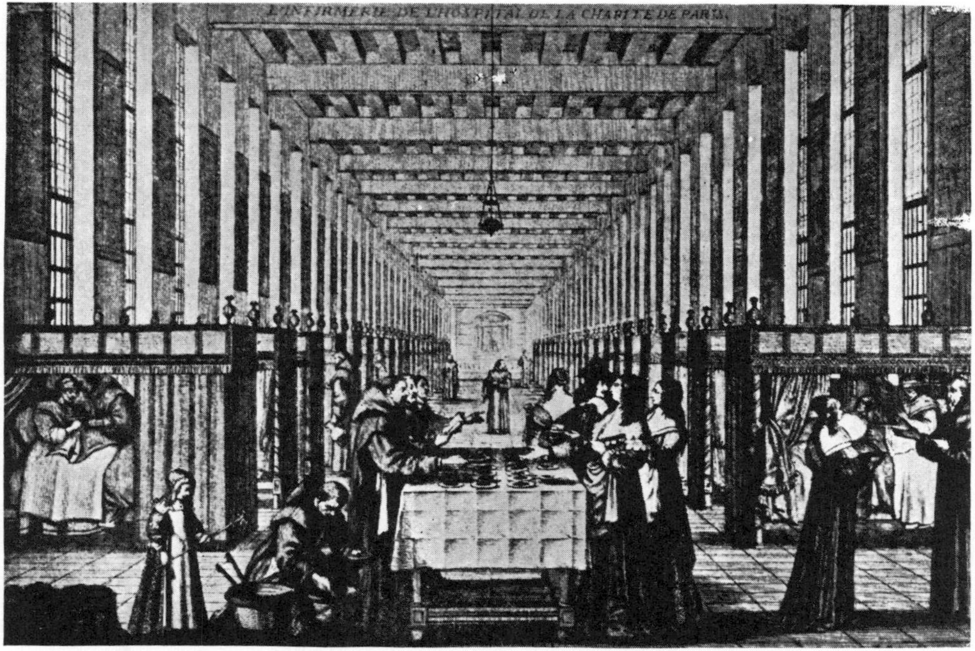

VIEW OF THE INTERIOR OF THE HÔPITAL DE LA CHARITÉ AT PARIS DURING THE REIGN OF LOUIS XIII
(*After an engraving in the collection of the Carnavalet museum*)

and even our profession, against which the letter of M. Sorbiére is full of atrocious insults.

Patin knew Pecquet personally and records several interviews which he had had with him.

Triaire quotes from Tallemant des Reaux an amusing anecdote about Riolan. He was cut for stone in the bladder but some time afterwards had a recurrence, for which he refused to be cut again. His wife concealed Colot, the famous lithotomist, in the house. One day Riolan said he felt much better and thought he could stand the operation, and that he believed he would have himself cut if Colot were at hand. Thereupon, Colot appeared, and Riolan exclaimed that he could not have the operation; that he was not ready as he had not confessed. "All will fall on us," said Colot, "we will be damned for you, but you will be cut." He tied him up and cut him and then said, "Confess now, if you wish to." "No," said Riolan, "I am too well for that."

Patin often speaks with great admiration of the skill of the famous family of Colot. There were three of them who attained great fame as lithotomists. Patin, writing to Falconet (May 13, 1659), speaks of Javot, also a lithotomist of note, but not in

Patin's good books, who had had the misfortune to lose three patients on whom he had operated. "The little Colot has cut many others who have recovered. I hope he will become as good and successful an operator as his father."

Patin writes Charles Spon (December 5, 1656):

> We had here two cousins who were very expert men at cutting for stone in the bladder, the younger named Gyrault died, aged fifty years last July, at Evreux, where he had gone to cut a gentleman. He had formerly cut the present Pope at Cologne. The other named Ph. Colot, aged about fifty-eight years, was a *peritissimus artifex.* He has gone to cut a man near la Rochelle, fell ill with dysentery, and died at Lusson. *Voila* today A. Ruffin formerly surgeon at la Charité the foremost lithotomist of Paris. There are yet others who run after this lucrative reputation, as Javot, surgeon to la Charité, Govin, of the Hôtel-Dieu, and another Colot, a cousin of the deceased, who was at Bordeaux, but has come here to search his fortune.

Stone in the kidneys or bladder seems to have been an exceedingly common complaint throughout Europe in the seventeenth century. Luther died of it, jestingly remarking that he was dying the death of Saint Stephen. Cutting for vesical calculus was a very common operation almost exclusively in the hands of a class of special operators known as incisors, among whom the most illustrious were the Colot family of whom Patin so often speaks. His own therapeutics in such cases was quite simple. In 1649 he writes Falconet, who was a sufferer, to refrain from wine, drink plenty of water, and be bled six times a year, and as often take a purge of cassia and senna with syrup of white roses. He tells him it is a disease of literary men, *litteratorum carnifex.*

Some charlatans pretended to cure stone in the bladder by secret remedies or methods, without the use of the knife. Patin[1] tells of one named Metiries, who claimed to dissolve the stone in the bladder by the injection of a certain medicament. He extorted enormous fees from his patients, claiming that his remedy was extremely expensive to make.

HONORS CONFERRED ON PATIN

When Riolan oppressed with old age and sickness, resigned his chair as professor in the Collège Royal, 1654, in favor of Patin, the

[1] Letter to Charles Spon, July 13, 1667.

latter writes Falconet (October 9, 1654) with pardonable pride and joy to tell him the good news. He is to teach botany, pharmacy, and anatomy.

I will direct all my care to make good scholars who should be far from the Arabs and the impostures of chemists, who are the ordinary persons by whom young physicians are today empoisoned.

I must make you the sharer in some good news with which you will not be vexed, that is if you do not pity me as one does sometimes those one loves, seeing that that which I shall tell you of will cause me much labor. It is that the goodman, M. Riolan, feeling that he had become old and nearly overwhelmed by a burden as heavy as Mount Etna, considered me above all others worthy to have his place as professor royal, and it has been fortunately accomplished. M. Amory, bishop of Coutances and grand Vicar to M. le Cardinal Antoine, grand aumonier de France, received and agreed to my nomination by M. Riolan. From them we went to M. de la Vrillière, secretary of state, who signed our letters; finally we carried them to the *gardes des sceaux*. M. Riolan alleged his reasons to which the former replied that he knew M. Riolan very well and his merit, and that he knew me also, that he would have them sealed next Monday, that we should be present, and he would gladly expedite us. Thus there only remain a few ceremonies to observe and to take the oath of fidelity at the hands of M. the bishop of Coutances.

Patin writes to Charles Spon (March 2, 1655) that he began his lectures with the following announcement "Guido Patin, doctor medicus et professor regius rei anatomicae et pharmaceuticae, clarissimi viri D. Jean Riolani, antecessoris sui, enchiridium anatomicum et pathologicum explicabit, ac alequot animadversionibus illustrabit. Initium faciet, die lunae 8 martii 1655, hora tertia pomeridiana in auditorio regio."

He describes (March 2, 1655) his introductory address:

It lasted a whole hour but it was not tiresome because it was a continuous history of the Collège Royal since the year 1529, when it was founded by François I, by whose successors the institution has been maintained, and governed by the grand aumoniers of France. Then I talked of the former professors who had rendered the Collège illustrious, such as Danesius, Turnebus, Carpentarius, the Durets, the grand Simon Pietre, and those who are yet living, as M. Riolan, to whom I testified my gratitude for having chosen me as his successor. I saw there some white monks and even four children of the fortunate Père Ignace, I know not how they came there without being invited. One of our physicians just told me he had returned from the College of Cambrai yesterday with one of our antimonial companions, from whom he demanded what he thought of my harangue. The doctor answered that the Latin of it was good, but that there was too much idle talk in it, that I had deceived him as he had expected that I would talk against antimony, but that I had said nothing about it.

Patin gave a sort of postgraduate course to his former scholars. He writes Charles Spon (September 16, 1650):

For my conferences for which I employ two hours one afternoon a week, they are good and can sometimes profit by some words on a question or controversy in medicine, but he (M. Sorbiére) lost his time when he attended them. I am under an obligation to him, as well as to the goodness of M. Duprat who did me the honor of bringing me such an auditor. If I had discovered or seen you there, you would have rendered me unable to speak as happened to Guillaume Bude before Emperor Charles v. They are little light interviews that I take pleasure in giving to my old scholars, to fortify them in the right method (of practice).

Writing (October 8, 1655) to Belin, *fils*, Patin tells him that during the week he had made a public dissection of the body of a woman who had been executed and that his demonstrations had been attended by a very large number of students.

In 1655 Patin was offered a professorship at Bologna, with a salary of 2,000 *écus*, and the opportunity of acquiring a large practice in that city. He declined, and writes Falconet (September 21, 1655):

> Neither ambition nor the desire to become rich shall make me quit Paris. Five years ago I declined to go to Sweden with much better conditions. I am cured of the *perigrinomanie* and the *philargyrie*, or rather I have never been sick with them.

In 1658 the Ambassador of Venice asked Patin to go to Venice promising him a salary of 6,000 francs a year from the Senate of the Republic, and the prospect of acquiring a large practice. Patin says that his name was suggested to the Ambassador by de Gorris, one of his pet aversions. He declined the offer on the ground of his health and his desire not to leave Paris. The Ambassador then offered to give the appointment to his son, Robert Patin, but

Guy would not hear of his accepting it, stating that it was necessary for his son to study five or six years more with him before he would be qualified to fill the position. He writes Falconet: "Italy is a country of syphilis, poisonings, and atheism, of Jews, renegades, and the greatest rascals in Christendom, all there is monkery and hypocrisy."

Patin received an invitation to go to Denmark. He writes Falconet (May 4, 1663):

M., the Prince of Denmark and M., his Ambassador, wish to take me from here, and bring me to that cold country. They have written to their King, and he has charged them to take me. They have made me beautiful offers, but I do not wish it. I am neither to be sold nor bought. I wish to be buried at Paris near my good friends.

The premier president of the court of the Parlement of Paris, Lamoignon, was a great personage, and Patin writes Falconet (May 20, 1659) with evident pride:

I supped last Saturday with *M. le Premier Président*, where he made great cheer. One eats quickly with him and talks little during the repast. He wished however, that I should drink his health twice in Spanish wine, which was extraordinarily good. Afterwards I talked with him a good hour and a half on various things in which he took great delight. He told me he was in difficulty how we should manage in the approaching summer, that he had wished to have leisure to talk with me once a week, an entire *après-dîner*, and that he feared, for lack of leisure, he would forget the little he had learned. Two *maîtres des requêtes*, who had come there to sup because of me, brought me away in their *carrosse*. He told me in parting that he had a design to make at his house a little academy, at least once a week, but he did not wish we should be more than six. He signified that I should be one and I believe my son, Carolus, will be of it also, because *M. le Premier Président* wishes as much good to him as to me.

It has been asserted, but without proof that the premier president used to have a louis placed under Guy's napkin each time that he was his guest. Patin, naturally, makes no mention of it, and the story seems to have been mere gossip.

Patin writes to Falconet (February 19, 1659):

M. le Premier Président sends for me sometimes to sup with him. He gives me great cheer, but his good welcome I value more than all the rest. I have promised to sup with him every

Sunday in Lent, and later we will take other measures, according to the season. There is much pleasure with him, because he is the wisest man of the long robe (lawyer) in France. He is very sage and very civil and says, smiling, that it is needless to speak evil of the Jesuits and the monks, nevertheless he is ravished when some *bon mot* against them escapes me.

Patin seems to have been a popular lecturer; at least his lectures were well attended. He writes Spon (April 21, 1655):

I gave my first lecture today in the great hall of Cambrai. I had fifty-two scholars who took notes, and some (other) auditors . . . The same day when I gave my second lecture at Cambrai I had by actual count sixty-two auditors. As I saw that they enjoyed listening to me, I made my exposition last an entire hour, and went forth amidst great applause.

In 1657 he writes Spon that his first lecture was attended by ninety persons and his second, by one hundred and fifty.

Patin was on terms of intimate friendship with Pierre Gassendi (1592–1655) whom he terms "an abridgment of all the moral virtues and of all the great sciences." He also calls him one of the most honest and learned men of the day in France. Gassendi was a priest and was chiefly distinguished as a philosopher and mathematician though he was also a good anatomist.

PATIN'S OPINION OF PHYSICIANS

Charles Saumaise (Salmasius) was a great source of admiration to Patin, who terms him that "excellent and incomparable personage" in a letter to Spon (October 26, 1643). Saumaise was born in 1588, and died in 1658. He was not a physician but a philosopher and theologian. Like most of the savants of his time he dabbled occasionally in medical matters. To English readers he is most familiar as the antagonist of John Milton in a pamphlet war, in which Saumaise supported the Stuart cause. He was a Huguenot, but nevertheless Richelieu sought to attach him to his services.

Patin was greatly wrought up by hearing the statement made that Saumaise had spoken ill of physicians, so he writes to Spon[2] that he has searched the writings of Saumaise to discover the place where he did so. He discovered that in writing of Attic and Roman law, Saumaise had referred to physicians as being mercenary. Patin says he is wrong to do so because on an occasion when Saumaise had been

[2] September 12, 1645.

ill in Paris, he had been attended by physicians who, after saving him from the hands of a charlatan into which he had fallen, had declined to accept any pay for their services to him. He attributes the statement made by Saumaise to the fact that he had lost three children in one year, of smallpox, while living in Holland, due, thinks Patin, to the "rude and gross" methods of practice among the physicians of that country.

He is astonished that Saumaise should have expressed such an opinion. He adds that he only augments the number of those who have done so, of whom Pliny is chief.

As to Michel de Montaigne, of whom I make great case, he has honored doctors personally by his approbation, and has only attacked their profession; and nevertheless he has been too hasty; if he had lived ninety or one hundred years before condemning medicine, he would have had some color of reason, but having been sickly from early youth, and having lived only seventy years[3] it is necessary to acknowledge that he paid the debt too soon; wise travelers only mock the dogs of the village after they are got to a distance, and when they cannot be bitten.

[3] Montaigne died when only fifty-nine. He was born in 1533 and died in 1592.

Patin's own cynicism about members of his profession is shown in the following passage:

> I will say, to the shame of my art if doctors were only paid for the good that they actually do, they would not gain so much, but we profit from the foolishness of women, from the weakness of sick men, and from the credulity of everybody.

Yet he writes Falconet (November 4, 1650):

> I will never speak insultingly of a doctor of medicine, because of the honor I bear to the profession, but I avow to you that all the chemists (Van Helmont, Guénault, etc.) that I have known until now have been poor vagabonds, boasters, braggarts, and liars, or very ignorant impostors.

Patin refers again to those who have written against physicians in a letter to Spon (October 19, 1649), mentioning that among those who had done so were the elder Pliny, Montaigne, and Agrippa. He says that in the month of February, 1617, the cold was so intense that his father and mother took him home from College, as they feared he would not be as warm there as by their fireside.

I remember that this little vacation was very agreeable to me, and being near a great fire much to my comfort, where the wood cost nothing, I read nearly all of a folio among the books of my late father, which was the "Commentaries" of Blaise de Montluc . . . He writes of pests and plagues, and declaims therein very rudely against the great number of physicians, advocates, and procurers, whom he calls the vermin of the palace . . . A gentleman named Rampole made here an academic discourse in which he extended himself greatly against the inutility of a very great number of men of letters in a state, wherein he spared neither physicians nor others. I avow veritably that there are in France too many priests, monks and ministers of chemistry, I mean procurers and lawyers of all kinds. I do not even doubt that in the country and in the small towns there are too many physicians, and that many of them are very ignorant. In Amiens, which is a small city desolated by wars and the passage of armies, there are today twenty physicians. But those of whom there are undoubtedly too many in France are the monks and the apothecaries, who cut miserably the purse and throat of many poor people. In recompense there are very few good and wise physicians who have been well educated and taught. I see them even here, *qui malunt errare quam doceri*, although they have good means to amend themselves. As to the country, it is overrun with miserable physicians, *qui de se nihil nisi magnifice sentiunt,* because they have dipped their noses in Perdulcis, of whom they only understand half the terms, or they have heard tell of diamargaritum, of apozemes, of cordial juleps, and of *vin émétique.* The principal cause of this misfortune is the too great ease with which the little universities make doctors. They give parchments too easily for money at Angers, Caen, Valence, Aix, Toulouse, and Avignon. It is an abuse which merits punishment since it redounds to the detriment of the public, but by misfortune we are not in a state of amendment . . . But perhaps God will finally have pity on us, and will change these things.

Patin was himself the object of several literary attacks. He describes to Charles Spon (January 6, 1654) a little book entitled "Bibliotheca Patinici," which was written in 1630 by Victor Pallu, a physician of Tours, in which he says he got off lightly but that some of the other physicians of Paris, notably Nicolas Pietre, Merlet and Moreau were very badly treated. The book was probably privately printed as Patin says that it was very rare. It was anonymous and Pallu's authorship was only discovered by the efforts of Moreau, who pardoned him at the intercession of his friends, though many other physicians bore him much ill will for his malicious attack. Pallu got into trouble also with his colleagues in Tours, so he left that city and went to Sedan, where he became physician to the Comte de Soissons. After the death of the latter in 1641, Pallu came to Paris where Patin says he dined with him twice. Patin speaks as though they were on perfectly good terms, though he says "the public lost nothing when he died," in 1647.

Patin in a letter to Charles Spon (September 17, 1649) mentions that he had heard that a physician of Montpellier, named Arnauld, was about to publish a book against him entitled "Patinus fustigatus." He says that this news neither astounds him nor surprises him, but that while he is obliged to wait for its appearance he would like to know something about its author, his quality, his age, and his object in writing, if he writes in defence of the chemists or the apothecaries or to refute Patin's thesis, or against his person and manners: "If he insults me I will let him alone and pardon him; if he says what is true and right so that I can learn something I will thank him; if he merits an answer I promise him one, provided that I have the leisure." Of course it should be remembered that none of Patin's letters had been published at this time.

On October 16, 1650 he again writes to Charles Spon that he hears that the book against him is to be a large quarto. "Each page is headed *Patinus verberatus*, a title manifestly satiric, insulting, scandalous and defamatory. I wish you would tell them that I believe that it is necessary to act against him and the printer, *nomine injuriam*, this title being purely defamatory. I am curious to know why this man is angry at me, and what wrong I ever did to him or his."

CONTROVERSY WITH RENAUDOT

Among the most interesting controversies in which Patin engaged was the famous one between Théophraste Renaudot, "the gazetteer," and the Faculté de Médecine. Renaudot presents an interesting character study as a quack whose intelligence led him to institute really big things, though it is very open to question, whether he himself realized their utility, and he certainly could not have anticipated their subsequent developments. Born at Loudun about 1586, he received the degree of Doctor of Medicine at Montpellier in 1606. He became acquainted with the famous Joseph François Leclerc, Marquis de Tremblay, more generally known as Père Joseph, a Capuchin monk, who was Cardinal Richelieu's right hand man and the only human being in whom he seems to have had implicit confidence. Renaudot went to live at Paris in 1612, with the strongest recommendations from Père Joseph to Richelieu. These led to the latter procuring for him the appointment of physician-in-ordinary to the King, Louis XIII. He became a favorite of Louis, and speedily procured the royal authority, backed by a decree of the Parlement of Paris, to establish a *bureau d'addresses*, or sort of employment agency, to which he added a pawnshop, or Mont-de-Piété, where money was advanced on the salaries of the borrowers, and also a free dispensary, or *consultations charitables*, all of which establishments are fully described in a pamphlet entitled "Inventaire de bureau de rencontre où chacun peut donner ou recevoir avis de toutes les nécessités et commodités de la vie et société humaine," published at Paris in 1620. The following year he began the publication of a newspaper, *The Gazette,* the first French newspaper.

Readers of Cyrano de Bergerac will recall the scene in the second act in the restaurant of Ragueneau, when the crowd is overwhelming Cyrano with congratulations on his victory over his hundred assailants at the porte de Vesle. He is approached by a "man of letters" with a writing case, who asks him if he can have the details of the contest. Cyrano repulses him, whereupon his friend, Le Bret, tells him: "He is Théophraste Renaudot! the inventor of *The Gazette.*"

> Cette feuille ou l'on fait tant de chose tenir!
> On dit que cette idée a beaucoup d'avenir!

Those of us who are interested in Guy Patin can only express our regret that the great French poet did not see fit to make him likewise a figurant with his antagonist.

He shortly afterwards ran foul of the Faculté de Médecine by attempting to establish, with the connivance and assistance of the doctors of Montpellier and the apothecaries, a rival school of medicine. The attempt was fraught with danger to the eminence of the Faculté, and they at once entered upon a fierce struggle with the audacious Renaudot, who, backed by the formidable friendship and favor of the King and Cardinal, put up a good fight. The death of Richelieu on December 4, 1642, was fatal to Renaudot's chances. In March, 1643, Patin wrote to Spon that "he had folded his baggage" since the death of his chief support. In the same letter he refers contemptuously to a recent publication of Renaudot's "La présence des absents, ou facile moyen de rendre présent au médecin l'état d'un malade absent. Dressé par le docteur consultant charitablement à Paris, pour les pauvres malades" in which he discourses on a method of treatment by correspondence which he had organized and which as Triaire remarks has certainly not been equaled by contemporary charlatans, nor, we might add, by the Christian Scientists.

Before his death, Richelieu had accorded to Renaudot a large amount of land in the faubourg St. Antoine, ostensibly for the *consultations charitables*, but Triaire states that the ground was really intended for the purposes of the school of medicine which Renaudot proposed to found in opposition to the Faculté de Médecine. The Cardinal hated the University of Paris because it possessed certain rights and privileges which were in opposition to the royal power,[4] by means of which its professors and students were often not amenable to the despotic power Richelieu wished to wield, Triaire thinks that the Cardinal backed Renaudot in his scheme with the deliberate purpose of destroying or, at least, lessening the power of the Faculté de Médecine. This explains the extreme animosity of the physicians toward Renaudot and the ardor with which they pursued the fight against him. The contest was not just with a successful charlatan, but against the despotism of the all powerful Minister, and it is little wonder that we find Patin breathing a sigh of relief

[4] Among other privileges claimed by the Faculté de Médecine of Paris, was that of exemption from military service. In 1634, the Spanish and German armies invaded France and succeeded in capturing Corbie, only thirty-three leagues from Paris. The country rallied patriotically. All the great bodies of the state subscribed to the fund raised by Paris, which also raised 28,000 men. The Faculté gave 1,000 *écus*. Patin writes to Belin, August 29, 1636, that the Faculté de Médecine claimed its exemption from military service on account of exemptions often confirmed in its registers. He adds that he himself has subscribed 12 *écus* to the fund raised by the Faculté.

at Richelieu's death, "il est en plomb, l'éminent personnage."[5]

In a letter to Spon (March, 1643) Patin again joyfully refers to the great man's decease. "The Gazetteer is living with Guillot le Songeur since the death of his inspirer (protocale) who held him up against us. But, God be thanked, he has folded his baggage."

> Il est en plomb, l'excellent personnage
> Qui a nos maux a ri plus de vingt ans.

Patin writes to Spon[6] some details of the last illness and autopsy of Richelieu. The Cardinal died on December 4, 1642, after

[5] This is a quotation from a rondeau written by Miron which Triaire gives:

"Il est passé, il a plié bagage,
Ce Cardinal, dont c'est moult grand dommage,
Pour sa maison. C'est comme je l'entends;
Car pour autrui, maint hommes sont content;
En bonne foi, et n'en voie que l'image,
Sous sa faveur il enrichit son linguage,
Par dons, par vols, par fraude et mariage,
Mais aujourd'hui, il n'est plus le temps,
Il est passé.
Or, parlerons sans crainte d'être en cage.
Il est en plomb, l'éminent personnage
Qui de nos maux a ri plus de vingt ans."

[6] December, 1642.

only six days of acute illness, though he had been very feeble and in poor health for a long time. During the preceding summer he had been in the south of France busied in suppressing the insurrection of Cinq-Mars. He returned to Paris in a litter on October 17th. While absent he had been operated upon for an abscess of the rectum. Patin says that a few days before Richelieu's death, in desperation he had submitted to the ministrations of a female empiric, who had given him horses' dung in white wine, and that another charlatan had given him a pill containing opium, because he did not think that the treatment by his regular physicians had been after the most approved manner. Triaire[7] quotes from a contemporary account of Richelieu's last days:

November 28th the Cardinal was taken with a violent chill and pain in the side. Bouvard summoned, bled him twice in the night of Sunday or Monday, but the patient spat blood and his fever increased. From Monday to Tuesday the pain having augmented, they practiced two new bleedings. Tuesday, December 2nd, a consultation was held at which it was decided to make a new emission of blood, and to have recourse to purgatives. The fever having

[7] Lettres de Gui Patin, Paris, 1907, footnote, I, 155.

redoubled in the evening they made two more bleedings. On Wednesday, December 3rd, an empiric of Troyes named Lefevre, was called in and administered a pilule which seemed to give a little relief. Finally, Thursday, December 4th, the seventh day of the illness, the Cardinal was seized with cold sweats, and died at noon.

At the autopsy the brain was found to be of unusual size.

It is curious how frequently autopsies were performed at that time. Patin's letters describe many of them. Pic[8] conjectures it was because of the frequency with which the deaths of prominent personages were ascribed to poisoning, but this seems doubtful as they were performed in many instances in cases where no such suspicion could have been entertained. This may have been the reason that the bodies of the Kings of France were always subjected to an official post-mortem examination, but would hardly suffice to explain the frequency of the examination of the bodies of private individuals.

Richelieu was a dangerous antagonist. The war was conducted chiefly through the medium of virulent pamphlets. As Patin writes to Belin in May, 1641, if "the Gazetteer," as he terms Renaudot, had not been

[8] Guy Patin, Paris, 1911.

sustained by his Eminence, the Faculté would have instituted a criminal process against him, but it would have been doomed to failure against such influence. Michel de la Vigne, Moreau, Riolan, Patin and other members of the Faculté wrote tracts in which Renaudot was excoriated and held up to contempt. Richelieu ordered them to cease.

Renaudot seems to have been particularly stung by the attacks of Guy Patin, who had termed him "nebulo" and "blatero," a nebulous braggart. He had Patin summoned before the *Maître des requêtes*, and it is sad but true that Guy only extricated himself from the charge of libel by asseverating that the terms as he used them were intended to be applied to Guy de la Brosse, the founder of the Jardin du Roi, and not to Renaudot. The latter, not to be thwarted, got a sister of de la Brosse, who was dead, to sue Patin before the *Juges de requêtes de l'Hôtel*. At the trial of the process Patin distinguished himself by addressing the court in his own behalf for hours, "with an eloquence, erudition, and esprit" which made the judges marvel.

They gave judgment for Patin on August 14, 1642, and needless to say he was greatly elated at his triumph. The Faculté proceeded actively against Renaudot, after he was deprived of his powerful protectors, the King and Richelieu. They took the matter up before the Châtelet, accusing Renaudot of practicing medicine illegally, and procured an order by which Renaudot and his associates were commanded to cease their enterprises. Renaudot appealed to the court of the Parlement of Paris, which august body on March 1, 1644, also rendered a verdict against him. Thenceforth, he passed into obscurity and no longer troubled the repose of the Faculté.

One method of expressing his contempt of Renaudot which Patin used, appears somewhat undignified as well as laborious. On September 17, 1643, Patin caused a Bachelor of Medicine named Courtois to sustain before the Faculté, a *thèse* which Patin had written, "Est-ne totus homo a natura morbus" (Do the maladies of man all come from nature?). It had a great success, six editions being printed. In a letter to Spon (December 24, 1643) he tells him that he has sent him a copy, and directs his attention to a passage where, in writing of diseases of the nose, he will find after the word *nebulones* the name of Renaudot, by taking the first letter of each word of the eight following. I give the transcription of the passage as illustrative of a far-fetched seventeenth century witticism:

Corruptum nasum sequitur corruptio morum; existo enim masonum genere, qui, ancidulo ore loquuntur, nebulones sunt, Ridiculi, Effranaei, Nefarii, Ardeliones, Vafri, Dolosi, Obsceni Turbulenti, mendaces, maligni, invidi, quadruplatores flagitiosi, infames, contumeliosi, faccinorosi.

Writing to Spon (1650) of his great admiration for the poems of Ovid (Ovidius Naso), he says:

Ovid was a *bel esprit* and I would willingly reread his works if I had the time. For his surname Naso it pleases me by the sympathy which I have for the big nosed, and the hatred I bear to the flat (*camus*) which are nearly all stinking and filthy, as "The Gazetteer," Théophraste Renaudot, against whom I gained the beautiful process on August 14, 1642. Thus I remember in going forth from the Palace (*palais de justice*) that day, I approached him, saying, "M. Renaudot, you can console yourself because you have gained in losing." "How then?" said he. "It is," said I to him, "because flat nosed when you entered here, you are going out with a foot more of nose."[9]

Renaudot responded to Patin's personalities by equally sharp replies. Because of the fact that Patin confined his therapeutic measures almost entirely to bleeding (*la saignée*), syrup of roses and senna, he was nicknamed "Doctor Three S's."

Renaudot refers to this in the following epigram:

> Nos docteur de la Faculté,
> Aux malades parfois s'il rendent la santé,
> Ont besoin de l'apothicaire;
> Mais Patin s'en dispense et, plein de dignité,
> Avec trois S les enterré.

Patin[10] tells how the Faculté scored on "The Gazetteer" in one instance. A rich old abbé, who was one of Richelieu's attendants, had been attended by Renaudot during an attack of gout. Renaudot gave him a powerful purgative which aggravated his attack. The abbé discharged him and put himself in the care of a member of the Faculté, who cured him. The old gentleman felt so grateful that he gave the Faculté

[9] The French have a proverbial expression applicable to one who is humiliated or chagrined that he has received *un pied de nez.*

[10] Letter to Spon, March 28, 1643.

10,000 *écus* towards rebuilding. Patin writes: "'The Gazetteer' from whom this prey has escaped has too good a heart to break over it, but however, I do not doubt that he is much vexed."

Renaudot was obliged to give up his *consultations charitables,* his project for a college of medicine and his pawnshop, but permitted to continue his *bureau d'addresses* and *The Gazette.* He died on October 25, 1553. His two sons, Isaac and Eusebius, both became members of the Faculté de Médecine, but only after a decree of the Parlement of Paris in 1642 had ordered their admission, which order was not complied with by the Faculté until 1647 or 1648. They continued to publish *The Gazette,* but before taking the oath required for the doctorate, were obliged to give up the *bureau d'addresses* and disavow the conduct of their father, in an oath taken before a notary.

CHAPTER VIII

Patin Experiences Opposition

THE PHYSICIANS OF PARIS VERSUS THOSE OF MONTPELLIER

In a letter to Belin (June 9, 1644) Patin, summing up his opinion of Renaudot, says:

> The Gazetteer could not confine himself to medicine, which he never practiced, having always sought to make his living by some other occupation such as schoolmaster, author, pedant, spy on the Huguenots, gazetteer, usurer, chemist, etc. The occupation he followed last was the practice of medicine, which he never knew; he is a braggart, and an ardelio, of whom the crest has been lowered by the decree which we, the Faculté de Médecine, have not obtained by our power but by the justice and goodness of our cause, which was founded on a policy necessary in so great a city against the irruption of so many barbarians who have practiced swindling here in place of medicine.

In a footnote, Triaire[1] points out that this passage refers to physicians who were not members of the Faculté de Médecine

[1] Lettres de Gui Patin, Paris, 1907.

of Paris, an especially large number being graduates of Montpellier, who came to Paris and tried to establish themselves there in practice. The provost of Paris decided on December 9, 1643, and his order was affirmed by the Court of the Parlement of Paris (March 1, 1644), that no one should practice medicine in Paris who was not a doctor or licentiate of the Faculté de Médecine of Paris or an *agrégé*. By an old decree of November 5, 1504, exception was made for those who were physicians to the King or royal princes, or the greater nobility, during such time as the Court was in residence in Paris or its environs. After its great victory over Renaudot, the Faculté became so assured of its power that it refused to register the physicians to the duc d' Orléans and the prince de Condé.

This apparent illiberality was not confined to the Faculté de Médecine of Paris. While the physicians of Montpellier were trying to exercise the right to practice their profession in Paris, in spite of the statutes of the Faculté, they, at the same time, were prohibiting the practice of medicine at Montpellier by outside physicians by virtue of an ordinance of Louis XII dating back to 1496.

In a letter to Spon (December 6, 1644), Patin accuses the Faculté at Montpellier of selling its degree of Doctor of Medicine, and says that many who have begun their studies at Paris, go later to Montpellier and purchase their degrees. He adds that he scarcely knows of an illustrious physician of Montpellier and humorously quotes: "parturiunt montes, nascetur ridiculus mus." He then states that their fame was due to their knowledge of Arabic medicine, Guy's pet aversion, and that any real knowledge they had was derived from Paris. "We have for antiquity the greatest number of physicians to the kings, and the greatest men who have most profited the public by the excellent writings which they have left us."

It is rather curious to find Patin mentioning the position of court physician as a distinction. "There were scarcely any illustrious physicians of Montpellier before Rondelet, who had studied at Paris and owed his learning to our schools." Rondelet is frequently referred to by Patin in terms of respect. He was an eminent anatomist who for lack of other available anatomical material, dissected the body of his own dead child before his class at Montpellier.

In the same letter Guy writes most venomously of two physicians of Montpellier, Héroard and Vautier. The former was first physician to Louis XIII, and from his journal, which has been preserved, concerning the health of the king, we learn he was a very wise and skilful man; but Guy says he lost no opportunity to hit at the Faculté, probably because that august body was always jealous of his position and anxious to belittle him. Vautier was first physician to Louis XIV and Patin says he prided himself on three things, namely; chemistry, astrology, and the philosopher's stone, "but one does not cure the sick by these beautiful secrets. Hippocrates and Galen are the beautiful secrets of our profession, which he perhaps has never read." Vautier had been physician to Mazarin, and Patin states his belief that he will never be made *premier médecin* to the king because Richelieu in the plenitude of his power had never dared have his physician, Charles, appointed to the king in this capacity. Patin was disappointed in his prognostication, for Vautier was appointed, as we have said, first physician to Louis XIV. Vautier had been first physician to Marie de' Médici and had great influence over her. He was imprisoned during the reign of Louis XIII for his participation in some of her conspiracies. Patin says, "M. Vautier condemns our Faculté sufficiently often. He says we have only bleeding and senna, and boasts of his having great chemical secrets. He gives antimony boldly in any illness, even to children."

Patin[2] expresses very fully his opinion of the superiority of the medical school of Paris over its ancient rival of Montpellier. He says that the two most famous physicians of Montpellier were Laurent Joubert and Guillaume Rondelet, both of whom wrote works on medicine which were merely compilations of their lectures, and that Rondelet's celebrated "Histoire des poissons" according to de Thou, was not even written by him but by Guillaume Pelicier. All the rest of the writings of the professors of Montpellier are merely foolish pedantic lectures, especially those of Rivière, in which there is much charlatanry: "They are a stinking marsh of ignorance and artful impostures." Patin excepts Varandeus from his condemnations.

But what comparison is there between all these men with Fernel, Sylvius, L. Duret,

[2] Letter to Belin, *fils*, September 7, 1654.

Tagault, the two Pietres, Jean Duret, the Jean Martins, E. Gourmelen, Baillou, the elder Gorens, who the late M. de Bourbon said was more learned in Greek than even Galen; with the two Riolans, with a Guillaume Duval, with the late M. de la Vigne, all prodigies of learning by their polymathy and incomparable men in their practice.

Patin refers frequently to the efforts made by the physicians of Montpellier to have their right to practice at Paris established. On September 12, 1646, he writes Belin that they have presented a request to the Council by Monsieur Vautier which was rejected, the Chancellor stating that the decree of 1644 was only a confirmation of the ancient privileges of the Faculté de Médecine, given after the parties to it had been heard in five public hearings, and that it must stand. Guy adds:

In other times foreign (not Parisian) physicians wishing to practice, called themselves chemists, spagyrics, Paracelsists, boasting to cure the worst diseases without bloodletting, and to possess great secrets against all sorts of diseases, but today, we see here very ignorant strangers and charlatans who have no shame, and brazenly state that they are physicians of the Faculté of Montpellier.

Many of Patin's letters are in the same strain and the repetition grows somewhat monotonous. Courtaud, dean of Montpellier, felt so aggrieved by the attack on the physicians of his school in the Renaudot controversy that he took up the latter's cudgels and wrote a most violent tirade against the Faculté de Médecine of Paris and against Patin. This gave rise to further replies on their part, one by Riolan.

OPPOSITION TO THE USE OF ANTIMONY

Patin's attitude as regards the use of antimony was not simply, as so often represented, a blind hatred of the remedy, or due solely to the fact that its use was popular. He writes to Spon (June 2, 1645) that he considers it (and we must say justly so) a very dangerous and pernicious remedy except in the hands of physicians who are both judicious and experienced and that it is rightly considered dangerous because its use has become widespread in the hands of barbers and quacks whereby many people have been killed.

This opposition to the use of antimony got Patin into trouble during his term of service as dean of the Faculté de Médecine. One, Jean Chartier, a member of the Faculté,

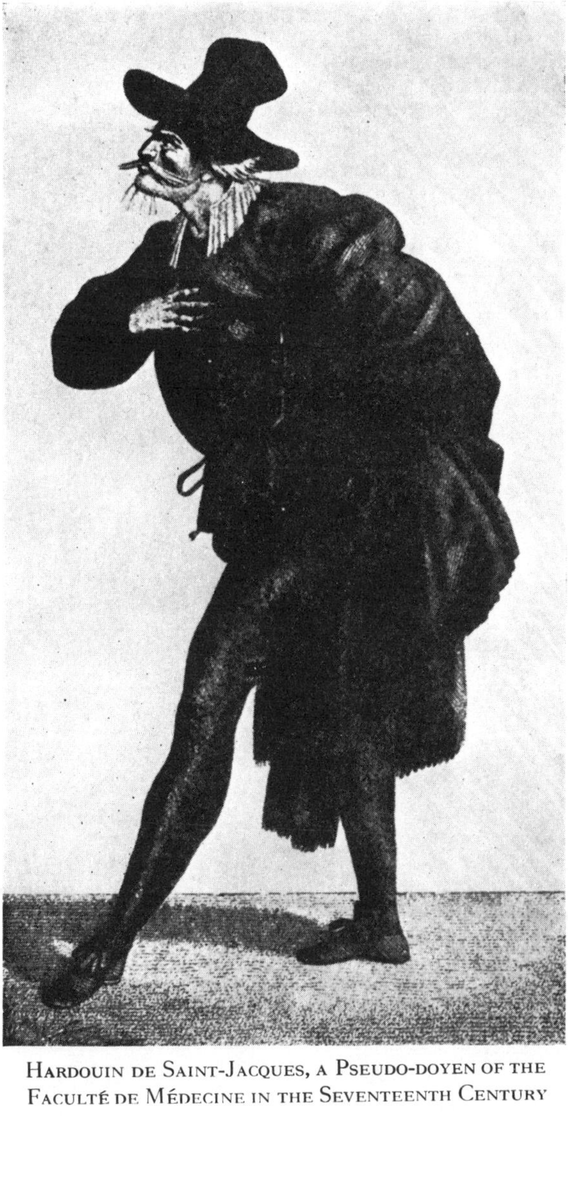

Hardouin de Saint-Jacques, a Pseudo-doyen of the Faculté de Médecine in the Seventeenth Century

having published a work advocating its use without having previously submitted it for the approval of the Faculté, Patin arbitrarily removed his name from the list of members of the Faculté. Chartier brought a complaint against Patin in the court of the Parlement of Paris. This august body having decided against Patin, reestablished Chartier in his membership, and condemned Patin to pay a large part of the cost of the process. This decree was rendered in 1653.

Patin wrote Spon (November 25, 1653) that judgment had been rendered against him through the influence of Guénault, and that the Queen had used her power to aid his enemies.

According to Bayle, Patin made a great register of those whom he claimed had died through the administration of antimony to them. He proposed to publish it under the title "Le martyrologie de l'antimoine."

It will be recalled that Molière in "Le médecin malgré lui" puts in the mouth of the young peasant, who comes to consult Sganarelle, the remark that an apothecary had wished to give his sick mother some *vin émetique* (antimony) but that he fears it will kill her, "as they say these great doctors kill I do not know how many people with that invention."

Patin[3] says that the controversy about antimony was largely maintained by the action of Hardouin Saint-Jacques, because without consulting the Faculty he had included *vin émétique* in his "Codex medicamentarius," and to sustain its inclusion had falsified the Registers of the Faculty for the year 1637, as had been publicly demonstrated by Merlet, Perreau, and Blondel, in spite of which Hardouin Saint-Jacques was never punished. In 1657 he writes Spon that Hardouin Saint-Jacques has broken his left arm by a fall from his horse: "It was he whose perfidy is the cause of all the disorder which has befallen our Faculty in regard to antimony, because being Dean in the year 1638, to favor the apothecaries, *a quibus lucrum sperabat,* he falsified the registers of the Faculty, but he has not heard the end of it." Hardouin Saint-Jacques according to Patin[4] had formerly been a comedian, having acted at the Hotel de Bourgogne.

Patin's correspondence contains innumerable references to the deaths of prominent

[3] Letter to Charles Spon, 1655.

[4] Letter to Falconet, December 19, 1660.

persons which he claims were due to antimony. A typical instance is one he details to Spon (December 6, 1650). M. d' Avaux, one of the superintendents of finances, was ill with some pulmonary trouble. Pietre, Seguin, and Brayer were treating him, but a relative (as sometimes happens even today) interfered and insisted that he should be seen by Vautier. The latter promised to cure him with a beverage he would give him.

The poor man swallowed the antimony on the good faith and standing of M. Vautier. An hour afterwards he commenced to cry that he was burning and that he saw that he had been poisoned, that he was sorry that they had allowed him to take the remedy, and that he regretted that he had not made his will. Then the poison having ravished his entrails, he died vomiting, three hours after having taken it.

According to Patin many said that Mazarin had had him poisoned as he was a bitter enemy of his. The day after Vautier was calling on de Maisons, the other superintendent of finance, when the latter said to him with pleasing candor, "*Voila,* two superintendents of finance that antimony has killed this year. I pray you do not make me the third." He referred to the deaths of d'Esmery and d'Avaux.

Patin in a letter to Spon (April 10, 1654) recounts: "Two days ago Guénault and des Fougerais gave their *Vin émétique* to a *maître des comptes* named de la Grange, who died of it. All this made much noise here at the expense of the reputation of these two executioners, who scarcely worry about it."

Antimony was usually administered as *vin émétique*. Patin in a letter to Spon (January 8, 1650) says: "*Vin émétique* is ordinarily nothing but an infusion of *Crocus metallorum* in white wine. As for the antimony goblet, it is more than twenty years since I have seen one, nevertheless the late M. Guénault had one which he used sometimes." Antimony cups or goblets, *pocula emitica*, had a great vogue in the seventeenth century. From the traditional origin of the name antimony one would have thought Patin would have been an advocate of its use. The metal, first known as *stibium*, was used as a medicine, especially by Paracelsus in the sixteenth century, but was introduced into wider medical use in a work entitled: "Currus triumphalis antimonii," purporting to have been written by a monk, named Basil Valentine, which was published in 1604. It is believed by most historians that no such person as Monk Basil ever existed, and that the name was chosen as a pseudonym by Johann Thölde, a Thuringian chemist. The author of the book alleges that he had observed that some pigs which had eaten food containing antimony, became very fat. He was led by this observation to try what its effect would be on some monks who had become very much emaciated as the result of prolonged fasting. *Horribile dictu!* They all died. Hence the name of *stibium* became replaced by the designation of *antimoine*, antagonistic to monks. Certainly if there is anything in a name Guy should have been an antimonialist of the most determined kind.

The history of the controversy about antimony is very curious and interesting. It raged at Paris for over one hundred years, dividing the profession into two camps, the antimonialists and the anti-antimonialists. It was waged not only in the conclaves of the Faculté but in the courts of law, and it caused the bitterest personal animosities and recriminations. After the publication of Valentine's book antimony became so popular and was used with such recklessness, that there were undoubtedly many fatalities from its improper administration. This led the Faculté to issue two decrees, in 1566 and in 1615, which were confirmed by the court of the Parlement of Paris, declaring antimony a poison and reprehending its administration. Notwithstanding these solemn denunciations many physicians in Paris, even members of the Faculté, continued to prescribe it. It must have been a sad blow for Guy when in 1666, the antimonialists finally triumphed, and the use of antimony as a medicine was formally admitted by the Faculté, and ordained by a decree of the Parlement of Paris. The vote repealing the decrees against it, and admitting it to the pharmacopeia was carried by forty-eight members of the Faculté, against eight. Poor Guy writes Falconet (July 30, 1666):

The cabal of the last assembly has wronged its reputation. These gentlemen say that a poison is not poison in the hands of a good physician. They speak against their own experience, because most of them have killed their wives, their children, and their friends. However that may be, they speak well of a drug which they dare not taste themselves. I console myself because it is necessary that there should be heresies so that the truth may be proved, but

I have never been of the humor to worship the golden calf, nor to consider fortune (wealth) as a goddess. God preserve me from it in the future. I am content with the mediocrity of mine. Peace and little! When the wind shall change, all these champions of antimony will scatter like the smoke from their furnace.

As would be expected from one of his temperament, Guy's opinions of his contemporaries are not always borne out by the facts we know concerning them. As an instance of this may be cited his violently unjust criticism of Julian Le Paulmier, one of the best known physicians of his time. Le Paulmier or Palmerius (1520–1588) received the degree of Doctor of Medicine at Paris in 1556, served four years as a physician to the Hôtel-Dieu, and was the student and friend of Fernel who bequeathed him his books and manuscript writings. Patin says he served Fernel as his "valet" for twelve years and that in recompense Fernel had him given the degree of doctor. In 1569 Le Paulmier published a book "Traité de la nature et curation des playes de pistolle, harquebuse et autres bastons à feu, ensemble les remèdes des combustions et brûleurs extrêmes et superficiels," in which, while agreeing with Paré in many of his views, he differed in others and even brought the charge that the great mortality among the wounded at the siege of Orléans and at the battles of Dreux and St. Denis was due to the methods of treatment employed by Paré and the other surgeons, thereby provoking a response from Paré. Although a Huguenot, Le Paulmier was physician to Charles IX and to Henri III and held by them in high esteem, as also by many of the great nobles of the court. He published two treatises on the medicinal use of wine and cider, and a number of consultations of his master, Fernel. In a letter to Spon in April, 1643, Patin calls Le Paulmier a wily Norman, adding that a Norman by race and a physician by profession possesses two powerful degrees to become a charlatan, and that he had bragged that Fernel had bequeathed him some very powerful secrets. He also accuses Le Paulmier of having, at a time when cider was not familiar as a beverage at Paris, brought up a quantity from Normandy and having put a little senna in it, sold it at a great price, as a wonderful secret remedy, thereby making a large fortune. Patin's hostility was possibly due to the great esteem in which he held Fernel and to a sort of jealousy of one who should have the right to be considered a favored disciple. Pierre Le Paulmier, Julian's nephew, published, in 1609, a book "Lapis philosophicus dogmaticorum," in which he advocated the doctrines and medicines of Paracelsus and the chemical school, at that time most vehemently combated by the Faculté de Médecine, for which he was suspended by his colleagues. Patin records somewhat vauntingly that "he continued in his chemistry, which suffocated him, having been surprised by an apoplexy near a furnace in the year 1610." Pierre Le Paulmier in turn left his papers to Théodore Turquet de Mayerne (1573–1655), the famous "chemical doctor" whose practices brought him under the ban of the Faculté de Médecine to such an extent that he was obliged to leave France and settle in London, where he became physician to James I, and after him to Charles I and Charles II, and achieved great fame and practice. Mayerne published at Geneva a book entitled "Enchiridion chirurgico praticum," which Patin says was undoubtedly composed from the papers Fernel had left Le Paulmier, which the latter bequeathed to his nephew, and he in turn to Mayerne.

It will be recalled that Mayerne, Guénault and others persisted in prescribing antimony after it was decreed by the Faculté de Médecine to be a poison and that the decrees of the Faculté had been solemnly authorized by the Parlement of Paris in 1566 and in 1615.

No words suffice to express Patin's detestation of Bourdelot (1610–1685), physician to Louis XIII and the Prince of Condé. Patin had been summoned to Sweden to act as physician to the notorious Queen Christina. He declined and Bourdelot went in his stead. Bourdelot is accused of encouraging the Queen in her vicious habits. Patin dwells especially on his avarice.

He disregards and always will disregard the Sunday Sermon to secure a quantity of gold.[5] He lies nearly as much as he talks, and when he can he deceives the sick also. He brags here in good company that he was the discoverer of the circulation of blood, and that his colleagues do all in their power to deprive him of the credit. He is a deep-dyed flatterer, grand servant of the apothecaries, and with all his fanciful bragging, a horrible liar.[6]

Patin adds that he had been apprentice to an apothecary and educated in his

[5] Letter to Spon, March 2, 1643.

[6] Letter to Spon, January 8, 1650.

father's barber shop. Bourdelot's real name was Pierre Michon but he assumed the name of his uncle, Edmund Bourdelot, physician to Louis XIII. Mazarin bestowed an abbey on him. Patin's bad opinion of him seems borne out by contemporary evidence although the language in which he expresses it is hardly seemly.

Patin's hatred of the Chartier family (three members of which were physicians, René, the father, and his two sons, Jean and Philippe) was intense. Jean Chartier, as told above, had been guilty of writing a book in favor of the use of antimony, and worse than that he had won in his legal action against Patin for reinstatement in the Faculté de Médecine. René Chartier was a very erudite man who devoted his life to the publication, in Greek and Latin, of a very commendable edition of the works of Hippocrates. When René died in great poverty Patin wrote to Spon (April 21, 1655) with exultation over his misfortunes, that "the widow is in desperate straits and Jean is living on the charity of the Bishop of Coutances." He was unable to pick any serious defects in Chartier's "Hippocrates" so he descended to a supercilious remark that it should contain a table of contents.

Guy's heart was never touched by compassion when his opponents suffered. Such misfortunes only seem to have added bitterness to his angry contempt for them.

A typical instance of Patin's attitude towards members of his profession whom he disliked, or rather hated, for it was not his wont to water his wine in such matters, is to be found in a letter he wrote Falconet (March 23, 1663), concerning a book written by Charles Bouvard (1572–1658). The latter was a brother-in-law of Riolan, *fils*, and had been physician to Louis XIII. He claimed that it was by following his advice and drinking the waters of Forges, that the long years of sterility of Anne of Austria were terminated, and that she gave birth to Louis XIV and his brother.

When a very old man he set himself to write a book for the reformation of medicine. The book was entitled, "Historiae hodiernae medicinae rationali veritatis ad rationales medicos," and was published in a very small edition at Paris about 1655. Patin wrote of it to Falconet on several occasions, telling him that Bouvard had shown advance copies to only three persons, Riolan, Moreau and himself. Patin thought very poorly of it. He says that though Bouvard was at one time an excellent man he was now senile, and that his life at the Court had corrupted him. He calls him elsewhere a dévout humbug, who would rather go to church twice than once. Patin writing some eight years after the publication of the book said that Bouvard was told by Riolan that he had better suppress the book as it contained matter which would anger Cardinal Mazarin and his two favorite physicians, Vautier and Valot. Bouvard accordingly withdrew from circulation the books that had been printed, Moreau and Patin both returning the copies he had submitted to them.

I know that he had talked to the late King (Louis XIII) of the merit and capacity of some of the doctors through whose hands the King had passed, until finally the King exclaimed, "*Hélas*, how unfortunate I am to have passed through the hands of so many charlatans!" These messieurs were Héroard, Guillemeau and Vautier. The first was a good courtier but a bad and ignorant physician. M. Sanche, the father told me in the past year that he was never a physician of Montpellier. The second was a wily courtier, who greatly desired to make a fortune, but the misfortunes of the Queen Mother, from whom he had hoped to receive it, carried him away, and the demon character of the Cardinal was stronger than his. So much so that he succumbed, and whatever effort he has made since, he has not been able to recover, although he has moved heaven and earth, and the late Prince of Condé himself spoke for him, even to Cardinal Richelieu himself, as well as to the late King and the Queen Mother. He had some good qualities, he also had evil ones. I associated with him twenty-seven years. We graduated at the same time. I knew well how he behaved. M. Baralis and I were his physicians until his death. Finally, I knew that in his practice there was much of hypocrisy and finesse; but also there was good doctrine and virtue, that is to say, of mixed merchandise. Vautier was an ignorant Jew of Avignon, very boastful and uneducated. He was fortunate not to have been hung, and he would infallibly have been so, if the poor Queen had lived six months longer. He had made counterfeit money, and subsequently found means to ensconce himself at Court. The disgrace of the Queen Mother gave him the entrée at Blois by the credit of Madame de Guercheville. He bragged that he possessed chemical secrets. . . . The Marillacs used him in their conspiracy against Cardinal Richelieu. The Day of Dupes[7] came.

[7] Journée des Dupes, November 11, 1630, thus called because on that date the Queen Mother and Richelieu caused the downfall of the conspirators who had been duped into believing that they were strong enough to overthrow them.

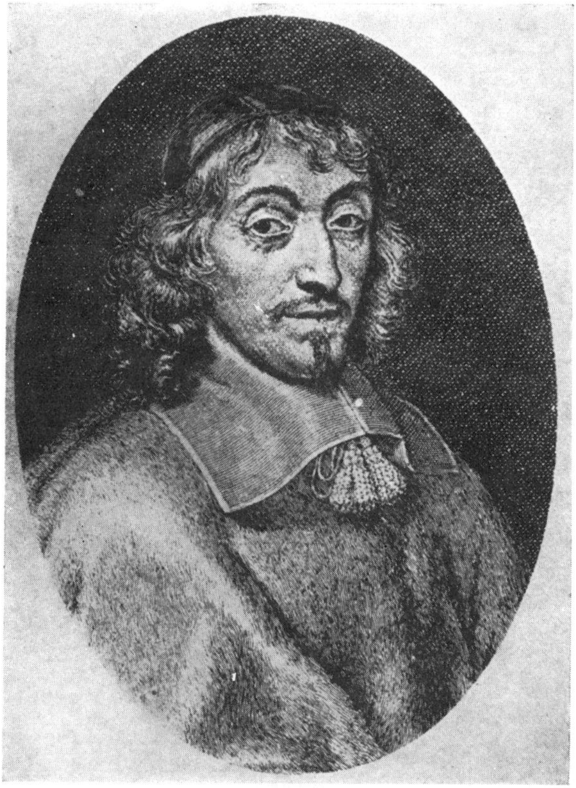

François Guénault
(15— –1667)

The Cardinal arrested the Marillacs and they were lost. Vautier was arrested and imprisoned in the Bastille for nearly twelve years. At length the scene and theater of the Court being changed, he became *premier médecin du roi*, by means of 20,000 *écus* which he gave to Cardinal Mazarin, who took from all hands, on condition, so they said, that he should be his spy. That is politics! He had been the father's prisoner for twelve years and they trusted him with the health of the son.

Another person who was most antipathetic to Patin was François Guénault, physician to Louis XIII, his wife, Anne of Austria, the Prince of Condé and many of the greatest personages of his time. He had probably the largest and most fashionable practice of any of the physicians of Paris, but he was a confirmed advocate of the use of antimony. He figures as Macroton, with the three other court physicians in Molière's "L'amour médecin." He was accused of being avaricious and unscrupulous. Patin writes of him that he was said to have stated "that one would not be able to extract the white crowns (*écus blancs*) from patients unless one deceived them." He elsewhere terms him "un grand empoisonneur chymique." Patin's hate poisoned his mind to such an extent that when Guénault's daughter died in childbirth, her father having administered antimony to her during her illness, Patin actually writes: "Guénault is a madman. By wickedness (*méchanceté*) he has poisoned his daughter."

Although a good friend of Patin's, Lamoignon did not employ him as his physician but had Guénault in that capacity. Patin writes Falconet (May 10, 1661) that he has been unable to secure an interview with the premier president for a townsman of Falconet's, because Lamoignon is ill:

He is in the hands of Sieur Guénault, who has retarded his recovery in place of hastening it, having purged him too soon, which obliged them to have recourse to bleeding many times. They have begun now to purge him but he has a severe headache which prevents one talking of any business to him. I have promised your friend that when he has recovered I will go and see him, and sometime I will try to obtain something for him. Do not be astonished that I am not his physician, Guénault has been so for more than twenty-six years, for political reasons.

When Guénault died, Patin wrote Falconet (May 17, 1667):

Today, in the morning, the 16th of May, M. Guénault died at St. Germain of an apoplexy

God did not permit that he should be saved by *vin émétique,* he, who in former times, has killed so many persons with this poison and with the *laudanum chymisticuni.*

On Van Helmont the judgment passed by Patin in a letter to Spon (April 7, 1645) was:

He was a wicked, Flemish rascal, who died insane a few months ago. He never did anything of value. I have seen everything he wrote. This man only thought of one method of practice, made up of chemical and empirical secrets. He wrote much against bloodletting, for the lack of which, however, he died in a frenzy.

In recent times the contributions of Van Helmont to medicine, especially to chemistry, rank much higher than those of Guy, or any of his contemporaries of the Faculté de Médecine of Paris. His investigations first directed attention to the fact that many of the processes of the living body were chemical and led to the chemistry of vital processes, and he discovered the chemical existence of gases, and their different natures, such as flammable and non-inflammable, noxious and innoxious, thereby opening up an entirely new field of chemical research.

Van Helmont, who was born in 1577 and died in 1644, was before Franciscus de le

Boë (1614–1672) the chief contemporary representative of the iatrochemical school, the founder of which was Paracelsus, consequently he was the living embodiment of evil to Patin's mind. Van Helmont's mystical theories of an archaeus, or governing principle of animal life, with a special archaeus presiding over each region or organ of the body made no appeal to Patin's materialistic mind, and he very rightly had no patience with the sympathetic ointment or powder, in support of which Van Helmont wrote a treatise. This sympathetic ointment, or weapon salve, was one of the most curious delusions which has ever prevailed in the medical profession. Briefly, it consisted in the belief that wounds could be healed by dipping something, preferably the weapon with which the injury had been inflicted, in the blood or discharges from the wound, and then dressing this object with the ointment or salve, applying bandages to it while leaving the wound itself undressed. In other words it was a form of "absent treatment." These ointments were variously compounded. Paracelsus, to whom is usually ascribed the start of the idea, especially recommended one composed of moss from a human skull, human fat and blood, mummy, oil of roses, bole armeniac, and linseed oil. Sir Kenelm Digby manufactured his sympathetic powder from a mixture of copper sulphate and other chemicals. When Patin hated once it was for good and all, and nothing which Van Helmont might do that was of worth could atone for his mysticism and chemistry. In justice to Patin it should be noted that most of Van Helmont's chemistry was but a dim foreshadowing of the discoveries of later days and it was so hidden in the jargon of mysticism in his writings that its significance is hard to find nowadays and must have been doubly so to his contemporaries.

Of the famous chemist Oswald Crollius, Patin in a letter to Charles Spon (February 20, 1654) wrote:

> I believe this man was never a physician, sage, or philosopher. He was a peculiar character, melancholy and ambitious, who, discontented with the ordinary science of the schools, wished to invent some other more certain. But he sought to fly without wings. . . . I have before heard the goodman Framboisière say that a German who knew Crollius had told him that this man was imbued with the desire to make two systems of science, one of theology, the other of medicine, without

any other authority than that of the Bible, and that he was usually hidden in a barn among charcoal and furnaces, under pretence of making chemical remedies, but that he was under suspicion of making there the false silver money, which is current in some parts of Germany. Is not that a fine occupation for a reformer of the sciences.

Guy de la Brosse, who was physician in ordinary to Louis XIII, was a skilful and learned man who founded the Jardin des Plantes, procuring patent letters for its establishment and being named its intendant in 1626. Patin wrote describing his last illness, in a letter to Belin (September 4, 1641): "He had a flux of the belly from eating too many melons and drinking too much wine. As to the last, it was not as much his fault as his custom." Patin tells how la Brosse took emetics, astringents and *eau-de-vie* but when bleeding was spoken of he said: "It was the remedy of sanguinary pedants and that he would rather die than be bled." "The devil will bleed him in the other world, as merits a rascal, an atheist, an impostor, a homicide, and a public executioner such as he was."

Triaire thinks possibly Guy's enmity was due to the fact that in founding the Jardin des Plantes this erudite naturalist took from the Faculté the privilege of teaching a very important branch of medicine.

Élie Beda des Fougerais, *premier médecin* to Louis XIV, who figures as Desfonandrès in Molière's "L' amour médecin," was, according to Patin,[8] not to be classed with honest men:

> He is a chemist, an empiric, and gains all he can by effrontery and impudence, without seasoning his actions with any prudence. He promises to cure everybody. He makes crazy statements of what he can do and of knowing more than anyone else; that such and such an one knows only how to bleed and purge, but that he possesses great secrets. . . . He was formerly a great giver of antimony but he did such poor business that he gave it up. . . . I do not like to talk nor think evil, but it is not through mischief that I speak thus of him, but in pure truth that you may know and recognize that this personage is a valet to the apothecaries and a grand cajoler of pretty women.

Patin writes of Beda's (the man's real name was Élie Beda, he added the des Fougerais of his own will) conversion to Catholicism to Spon (May 8, 1648) that it had "pleased God to touch the heart (I do

[8] Letter to Spon, August, 1650.

not say the soul because I doubt if he has one), of our master Élie Beda . . . He goes henceforth to mass, carries a chaplet, and acts the bigot, as the others."

On Joseph Duchesne (1521–1609) more generally known by his Latinized name Quercetanus, Patin pours forth the following diatribe in a letter to Spon (January 8, 1650). Quercetanus had been physician in ordinary to Henri IV and was an ardent follower of Paracelsus and an antimonialist:

> The same year there died here a wicked rogue of a charlatan, who killed many during his life, and also after his death by the miserable writings which he left under his name which he had caused to be made by other physicians and chemists from here and there.
>
> It was Josephus Quercetanus, who called himself at Paris the *Sieur de la Violette.* He was a great quack, a heavy drunkard, and one plainly ignorant, who knew nothing of Latin, whose first trade was that of surgeon's apprentice in Armagnac, which is a poor country. He passed at Paris, and chiefly at the Court, as a first-class physician, because he had learned something of chemistry in Germany.

Patin's hatred of the Arabic school of Medicine is fully explained in a letter to Spon (May 29, 1648) in which he writes that all that is good in their doctrine came from the Greeks. As to their remedies the school flourished at a time when they were in possession of better remedies than those known to Hippocrates but the Arabs made bad use of them.

The miserable Arabesque pharmacy was introduced and the rascally hot remedies, useless and superfluous, which are today in too much credit all over the world, and by a quantity of which the sick are villainously deceived. What good are all these compositions, all these sugared and honeyed alteratives, against which the wisest men in Europe have declared and raised themselves for a hundred years, as against an insupportable tyranny? . . . The great abuse of medicine is due to the multiplicity of useless remedies and the neglect of bloodletting. The Arabs are the cause of both. . . . We save more sick people with a good lancet and a pound of senna, than the Arabians can with all their syrups and opiates. We would do very wrong to quit the good remedies, which have come into use from the time of Hippocrates, for those which are less good or unknown to us. The method does not comprehend the remedy but the law and manner of using it rightly. It is the doctrine of indications which shows a physician as he really is, and for this we owe our entire obligation to the Greeks, who if they knew not senna and cassia it was not their fault, but their misfortune. Also it was not by the Arabs that senna was discovered and made known to us, it was in use before them. Strong and violent remedies are yet good for some, but the science and method of the Greeks teach us to use most successfully the benign and to keep away from those capable of harm, if we have not great need of them.

There is a brutality in Patin's references to those whom he hated, which is either a childish affectation or else an indecency. He writes to Spon (March 8, 1644) as follows:

> M. Merlet, eight days before the death of M. Richer, made a false step in mounting (his mule or horse) by which he thought he had broken his leg, but he only had a slight dislocation of the *péroné* (ankle). The wags say that he would have done better if he had broken his neck. That will be for another time when it will please God to deliver our school of this terrible fool.

MOLIÈRE AND PATIN

Guy's great therapeutic standbys were purgation, with senna or manna, enemas, and venesection. Some of his letters remind one forcibly of the chorus of the bachelors of medicine in "Le malade imaginaire" of Molière:

> Clysterium donare,
> Postea saignare,
> Ensuitta purgare.

A maxim of Patin's was "Marcher la saignée devant la purge."

Probably the ideas of most readers of the present concerning the medical profession in France during the seventeenth century are derived from Molière, wherefore it is well that we should stop for a moment to consider somewhat his attacks on them.

Three of his comedies are especially virulent in their attacks on the profession, "L'amour médecin," "Le médecin malgré lui" and "Le malade imaginaire." In "L'amour médecin" he caricatures a consultation between four of the King's physicians, Daquin or Valot under the name of Tomès, Élie Beda des Fougerais as Desfonandrès, Guénault as Macroton, and Esprit as Bahis, in such a way that his audiences, largely composed of courtiers must have hugely appreciated the joke, and readily recognized the originals under the scanty disguise.

It is said that Boileau suggested to Molière the names under which certain well-known characteristics of the physicians were revealed. Thus, Desfonandrès means "slayer of men"; Bahis indicated one who stammered; Macroton, a slow talker, as Guénault was known to be; Tomès, a bleeder, was applicable to Daquin, who was famous for his propensities in that direction. Elsewhere I have given Patin's own expressions concerning Guénault and des Fougerais. No ridicule which Molière could throw at them could equal the contempt which Patin, their colleague, heaped upon them. Patin writes to Falconet (September 22, 1665):

They performed a short time ago at Versailles a comedy about the physicians of the Court, in which they were treated with ridicule before the King who laughed at it very much. They put in the chief place the first five physicians, and above all our master, Élie Beda, otherwise the Sieur des Fougerais, who is a man of great probity and very worthy of praise, if one believes that of which he would persuade us.

A few days later, September 25, 1665, Patin refers again to the performance of "L'amour médecin." "They are now performing at the Hotel de Bourgogne, 'L'amour médecin.' All Paris crowds there to see represented the physicians of the Court, chiefly Esprit and Guénault, with masks especially made. They mock those who kill people with impunity."

Patin does not state that he himself saw the play. He writes to Falconet (March 29, 1669) that all Paris is going to see "Tartufe." Reveillé-Parise thinks that the austerity of the manners of physicians rendered it customary for them not to go to the theater.

There is no doubt that the members of the Faculté de Médecine of Paris in the seventeenth century laid themselves open to the shafts of ridicule. It was a close corporation holding tenaciously to ancient privileges, admitting to its membership only a chosen few each year and those chiefly drawn from the ranks of relatives and friends of those already members. In its very reaction against the poor tradition of Arabic medicine, the relic of medieval barbarism, towards the pure Greek tradition, it did not escape from slavish subservience to the latter, and at a time when many were escaping from dogmatic adherence to ancient forms and rebelling against submission to authority simply because it was ancient, the Faculté tried in vain to stem the current. Molière combated hypocrisy and affectation wherever he found them and these two vices were preeminently displayed by members of the Faculté. Molière's health was poor and he had to have recourse frequently to medical aid during the later years of his life. He had as his physician Mauvilain, whom he seems to have respected, and for whose son he besought the only favor he is known to have asked of the King, an ecclesiastical preferment. It is true that when Louis XIV asked him how he and Mauvilain got along with one another, he replied: "Sire, we talk together; he prescribes remedies for me; I do not take them; and I recover." Probably his frequent intercourse with physicians and their inability to cure him caused his satirical ridicule of them in his plays. He died from a pulmonary hemorrhage and most probably had tuberculosis for many years before his death. Molière's only reference to Patin is somewhat indirect. During the consultation in "L' amour médecin" the doctors, not talking at all about the patient whom they have been called to see, discuss the quarrel between Théophraste and Artémius, the latter undoubtedly being Patin, and the other his opponent Renaudot.

Patin certainly read if he did not witness the comedies of Molière. In a letter to

Falconet (August 28, 1669) he uses the name Tartufe as synonymous with hypocrite. A physician named Cresse became involved in a scandal with the wife of a barber and Patin, writing to Falconet in 1669, in several letters says that it is reported Molière will write a comedy about the affair, but the great dramatist never did.

In many of his comedies besides the three mentioned above Molière indulges in sly hits at the medical profession. It is possible his ridicule did some good but there was no apparent great reformation in French medicine until shortly after the Revolution when there arose the great school represented by such names as Bichat, Laënnec, Trousseau, Louis, Dupuytren, Desault, Larrey, etc., which during the first part of the eighteenth century gave to their country the foremost position in medical science in the world.[9]

Patin was not a frequenter of the "theater-ballet" at the court, and he makes no mention of his ever having gone to see a play or having read one himself. The theater-

[9] Brander Matthews in *Appleton's Magazine*, August 8, 1874, and in *Scribner's Magazine*, January, 1910, has written most entertainingly of Molière and the medical profession.

going population at Paris was largely confined to the nobility or to the frequenters of fairs. Mauvilain, Molière's physician, was a classmate of Robert Patin's. Guy Patin refers to him occasionally in his lists of evildoers who gave antimony, and whom he accused of being avaricious for fees.

Patin only mentions Corneille once when, in a letter to Falconet (October 21, 1653), he tells him: "M. Corneille, the illustrious maker of comedies, is going to write an answer to Pellisson's 'Histoire de l' Academie.'"

Patin knew La Fontaine, the author of the celebrated fables. He writes Charles Spon in August, 1658, that he had shown La Fontaine a letter that Spon had written, and that La Fontaine had asked him to send him his good wishes.

BLOODLETTING

Patin's letters are full of references to the beneficent effects obtained by copious bloodletting, applied to diseases of the most infinite variety. A few extracts will suffice to illustrate his views. He writes to Spon, April, 1645, thus:

There is no remedy in the world which works as many miracles as bleeding. Our Parisians ordinarily take little exercise, drink and eat much, and become very plethoric. In this condition they are hardly ever relieved of whatever sickness befalls them if bloodletting does not proceed powerfully and copiously, nevertheless if the sickness is acute one does not see the effect as soon as from purgation. About the year 1633, M. Cousinot, who is today first physician to the King, was attacked by a rude and violent rheumatism, for which he was bled sixty-four times in eight months, by order of his father, and of M. Bouvard, his father-in-law. After having been bled so many times they commenced to purge him, by which he was much relieved, and in the end recovered. The idiots who do not understand our profession imagine that there is nothing to do but to purge, but they deceive themselves because if bleeding copiously had not preceded it, to repress the impetuosity of the vagabond humor, to empty the great vessels, and to chastise the intemperance of the liver which produced the serum, the purgation would have been useless. Another time I treated in this city a young gentleman of seven years, who fell into a pleurisy by overheating himself when playing tennis, having also received in the game a stroke on the foot on the right side, which provoked the most grand fluxion. His tutor hated bloodletting very much and I could only oppose to this hatred a good counsel, which was to call two of our ancients, M. Seguin and M. Cousinot. He was bled thirteen times and was cured in fifteen days, as if by a miracle, even the tutor was converted by it.

In the same letter he writes:

It is perfectly true that bleeding is a very powerful remedy in smallpox, especially if done early, but this disease is sometimes so insidious, and the lungs sometimes so involved that it is folly to promise relief from it. That is why prognosis is in this case so useful to the physician. It is my custom to say to mothers who generally have a great concern for the faces of their children, that it is necessary first to be assured of their life, and that I cannot answer for the outcome of this dangerous disease until after I have seen the children out in the street many times playing with other children.

Patin considered bleeding as the only therapeutic measure of any avail in apoplexy. He writes to Falconet (May 10, 1661): "This afternoon I gave a very good lecture in which I amply explained apoplexy, and belabored the apothecaries who would exhaust their shops on this malady, but in vain. We only cure it by prompt bleedings."

Patin again writes to Falconet (October 14, 1664) his views regarding the treatment of epilepsy. He begins by declaring his belief that there was no specific for it:

I believe that there are no anti-epileptic remedies. M. Seguin, Riolan, de la Vigne, and Moreau, are of the same opinion. Those which Crollius and the race of chemists vaunt as such, are fictions or fables. I do not except mistletoe, the foot of the eland, the root of peony, nor other similar bagatelles. The cure of such a great disease depends on an exact regimen of life, with abstinence from women, wine, and all hot and vaporous foods; but bleeding and frequent purgation are necessary. These do not hurt the brain, and are not made with pills or powders. It is necessary, sometimes also to evacuate the pus which is in the mesentery, the lungs, the hollow part of the liver, or the uterus, and the fits will not cease until such humor is evacuated. Fernel was a great man who broke the ice on many points, but he lived too short a time to know and tell all. He only lived fifty-two years. Pearls are of no use in it (epilepsy) except to enrich the apothecary.

Speaking of the desperate illness of M. Merlet, Patin tells Belin: "M. Merlet has been nearly at the gate, but he has not passed through the wicket." It is wonderful that he escaped because Patin tells us that he was extremely sick "of an inflammation of the lungs for which he was bled sixteen times in January. In a previous month, July, he was bled eighteen times for a malignant fever. Merlet was at that time sixty-six years old."

Patin was a "Brissotin," or disciple of Pierre Brissot (1478–1522) as one would naturally expect. Brissot brought into vogue "derivative" bleeding, that is bleeding from the side of the body on which the lesion was located, as taught by Hippocrates. To this was opposed the Arabian theory of "revulsive" bleeding, or drawing blood from the opposite side to that of the lesion. In support of this he writes to Belin, *fils* (March 14, 1649) after his father had had a paralytic stroke, urging that he should bleed him from the unparalyzed arm, or possibly a little later from the palsied one. Brissot's theory was applied especially to bleeding in cases of pleurisy.

For the benefit of the lay reader it should be stated that in paralysis due to an apoplectic stroke or hemorrhage in the brain the paralysis occurs on the opposite side of the body.

Brissot's teaching at a time when the Arabian school was at the height of its power raised such a storm that he was banished from France by the Parlement of Paris. The echoes of the controversy still lingered in Patin's time.

CHAPTER IX

Patin's Later Years

SURGEONS AND BARBER-SURGEONS

To the barber-surgeons, Patin was more lenient than to the apothecaries because the barbers were more humble in their attitude toward the physicians. Patin writes to Belin (January 14, 1651):

As for the barber-surgeons, they are only received with our approbation and after examination in our presence, and they are only permitted to practice surgery, not at all pharmacy, above all not to administer any purgative or narcotic except on the prescription of a physician.

"When each follows his *métier*, the cows are better watched." We have here very subservient (*souple*) surgeons. Bleeding makes them rich, but they know very well that they are in our hands and their gains also. They cannot admit candidates to their society (*Ils ne font point d'actes*) unless the dean of our Faculté is present, accompanied by two doctors who have the right to impose silence when they are extravagant in their questions, these three even have to sign the act of reception (of the candidate) otherwise he has not the right to open his shop. For the rest they love us as their patrons, they see how we have treated the apothecaries, and how we have nearly annihilated them, and that it would not be difficult for us to do the same thing to the surgeons, if they were not *souple* and did not rule themselves wisely towards us.

To Spon he writes (April 21, 1665):

I assure you that at Paris we hate the surgeons as much and perhaps more than the apothecaries, seeing that they are equally insolent, added to which they are companions of the country of *adicusias*, who promise marvels to poor people *quos impura Venus ut plurimum momordit.*

The history of the long quarrel between the physicians and surgeons of France has been accurately and thoroughly discussed by Malgaigne in the introduction to his edition of the works of Ambroise Paré.

In Patin's time there existed three classes of those who practiced the healing art; the physicians, the surgeons, and the barber-surgeons. The physicians, represented by the Faculté de Médecine, had formerly had control over both the surgeons, whose organization was known as the

Collège de Saint Côme, and the barbers who belonged to the society of the barber-surgeons.

In 1657 the barber-surgeons decided to amalgamate with the Surgeons of Saint Côme, frequently called surgeons of the long robe, because they wore a long robe similar to that in vogue with the physicians of the Faculté. This would have the effect of removing the barber-surgeons from the control of the Faculté and would strengthen the hands of the surgeons in their frequent contests with the latter. The surgeons had for centuries been ground between two millstones, the Faculté, which would not permit them to prescribe and regarded them simply as mechanical assistants to be called in when they were needed, and the barber-surgeons who were constantly trespassing on the surgeons' field and had for many centuries done much more and better surgical work than the surgeons of the long robe. The latter treated abscesses and wounds by the application of plasters and ointments, but most of the operative work was done by the barber-surgeons, from whose ranks the incisors, bone-setters, and lithotomists were drawn. Thus Franco, the Colots, and Paré himself were barber-surgeons, and there is no name of note found among the surgeons of Saint Côme over a period of some hundreds of years. Paré was only admitted to their ranks through the exertion of the King's influence after he had become famous, and in the face of great opposition on the part of many of the members.

Patin as might be expected was furious at the prospect of this union. He writes to Spon (July 13, 1657):

We are now at law with our barber-surgeons who wish to unite with the surgeons of Saint Côme, our ancient enemies. *Cosmiani illi* (those of Saint Côme) are miserable rascals, nearly all tooth-pullers and very ignorant, who have attached the barber-surgeons to their string, by making them share their halls and their pretended privileges, among others holding their examinations in their hall, wearing a long black robe and a square bonnet, and they demand that we be present at these functions, I mean our Dean, who goes there accompanied by two doctors. . . . They talk of (giving) degrees of bachelors, of licentiates and other such ceremonies and vanities, altogether indecent for such booted lackeys. The cause will be plead in a month and I believe that all the audacious designs of this superb mob will be bridled and regulated, and meanwhile our Dean will not be present at any of their functions. Are these surgeons of Saint Côme not agreeable? They had permission from the king about three hundred years ago by which they were given license to assemble together. They claim from this word license that they were permitted to make licentiates in surgery, which however they have never undertaken to do heretofore. . . . And they would make for us, doctors *pas latins* (ignorant of Latin), who would not know even how to read or write. We do not attempt to prevent them from being surgeons of Saint Côme, or that the others might unite with them, we would only have a company of barber-surgeons, as we have had until now, which would be dependent on our Faculté, and would take every year an oath of fidelity in our schools at the hands of our Dean, *in magnis comitatis Facultatis*, and pay us every year a certain sum for the rights which we have in their functions. But we do not wish robes, bonnets, licenses, nor any similar abuses. . . . They are already sufficiently vainglorious and stupid without furnishing themselves with any such apparatus.

The union was brought about in spite of the Faculté's opposition, to the great benefit of French surgery..

The legal proceedings were not terminated until 1660 in which year Patin wrote several letters to Falconet expressing his satisfaction with the terms of the settlement. They were satisfactory to Patin because, although the surgeons of Saint Côme and the barber-surgeons were united in one guild, it was placed under the authority and control of the Faculté de Médecine. This decree of the court was confirmed by another in 1676, four years after Patin's death, wherein it was ordered that the officers of the guild should appear each year, on the day after the feast of Saint Luke at the Écoles de médecine, to take the customary oath, pay a gold *écu*, and present a catalogue of their maitres to the deans of the Faculté. This distinction between the physicians and surgeons in France continued until August 18, 1792, when the Assembly abolished all faculties and corporations. After the Revolution, 19, *ventose an* XI, the medical schools were legally reorganized but the educational requirements were the same for the practice of either medicine or surgery and only one degree, that of M.D., was given to the graduates.

THE APOTHECARIES

A very famous victory was won by Patin in 1647, over those whom he called "mes chers ennemis," the apothecaries of Paris. The apothecaries had sided with Renaudot in his memorable attack on the Faculté de Médecine because of the condemnation by it of the use of antimony and its attitude against the Arabian polypharmacy which was such a great source of revenue to the pharmacists. Patin was especially conspicuous in the Faculté and both in speech and writing lost no opportunity to belabor the apothecaries for what he called their swindling and avariciousness. The new pharmacopœia published by the Faculté de Médecine was calculated to hurt the apothecaries very much as it had a distinct tendency to lessen the complexity of compounds and to encourage the use of the simpler preparations. Patin wrote a thesis "Estne longae ac jucundae vitae trita certaque parens sobrietas." This may be briefly summed up as "On Sobriety" and he caused it to be sustained by one of his scholars, Montigay, March 14, 1647. In it he poured out a long diatribe against the apothecaries, their methods and their preparations. The apothecaries brought an action in the court of the Parlement of Paris against Patin. Patin in a letter to Falconet (April 10,

1647)[1] tells how, acting as his own lawyer he discoursed for an entire hour, at the end of which the Court gave judgment in his favor and the apothecaries were driven from the hall, amidst the jeering and hooting of the audience, which according to Patin amounted to six thousand persons.

His description is so picturesque or Patinesque, that I transcribe it in full:

For my dear enemies, the apothecaries of Paris, complained of my last thesis to our Faculté which mocked them. They appealed against it to the Parlement, where their advocate having been heard, I myself responded immediately (*sur le champ*) and having discoursed an entire hour to a very large and very favorable audience (as I had also done five years ago against the Gazetteer), the poor devils were condemned, hooted, mocked, and confounded by all the court, and by six thousand persons, who were ravished to see them refuted and over-

[1] André Falconet (1612–1691) was a native of Roanne. He received his doctor's degree at Montpellier and practiced medicine at Lyons. He is first mentioned by Patin in a letter to Spon, April 21, 1643, wherein he asks Spon for information about a "M. Falconet who has written on scurvy" referring to a work by Falconet entitled "Moyens préservatif pour le guérison du scorbut," published at Lyons in 1642.

thrown as I had done. I talked against their bezoar, their confection of alkermes, their theriac, and their compositions. I made them see that *organa pharmaciae erant organa pallacae,* and made them acknowledge it to all my auditors. The poor devils of pharmacists were put to such confusion that they did not know where to hide themselves. All the city knew it and likewise mocked them, so much that honor came to me from all sides, the same as from our Faculté which rendered me thanks because I had so well defended myself from the annoyance (*pince*) of these good men, and in such a way that it went to the honor of our company. The judges even have praised me. *Voila, monsieur, l'histoire des pharmaciens.*

Paris really was a hotbed where all kinds of charlatanry flourished in Patin's time as is apt to be the case in any great city, and there was much cause for complaint. He writes to Spon (April 21, 1655):

There arrive here a thousand misfortunes because of the too great credulity of the sick, who address themselves to the surgeon's apprentices, apothecaries, charlatans, operators and other ignorant animals eager for gain. Note that the greater part of these strollers are Provençals, Languedociens, and Gascons, or from the neighboring provinces. This only occurs here because of the lack of police and negligence of our judges.

Patin was a vehement, not to say venomous, enemy when aroused, but also a very difficult one to combat, because of the careful preparations he made for his various combats and the skill with which he armed himself. Thus he writes to Belin (August, 18, 1647) that he is going to prepare for a future possible attack by the apothecaries, a work in which he will "refute the bezoar, the cordial waters, the unicorn's horns, theriac, the confections of hyacinth and alkermes, the precious fragments and other arabesque bagatelles," but that it will require three or four years of leisure to complete the book. In the two speeches which he delivered at the Renaudot trial and in his own defense against the apothecaries, his audiences were overpowered by his display of learning and the scope of the arguments with which he supported the sharp and witty invectives which he launched against his foes. Patin would surely have pleased Dr. Johnson as a "good hater." He certainly had the courage of his convictions. Writing to Belin (January 18, 1633) in speaking of the warfare the physicians were waging against the apothecaries because of avarice and extortion, Patin says:

In the majority of the grand houses there are no longer apothecaries, it is a man or a chambermaid who makes and gives the enemas, and the medicines also, which we have reduced to the laxative juice of prunes, or bouillon and senna with juice of citron, or orange, or verjuice, or a laxative ptisan of cassia and senna, according to the taste of the patient.

In a long letter to Spon (June 18, 1649) Patin bursts forth against the monks whom he hates almost as bitterly as the Jesuits. After a long tirade he writes:

But leave that pest of religion to pass to that of medicine, I mean the apothecaries. You (the physicians of Troyes) have made an agreement with them; they are not worthy to enter into a composition with their masters, upon whom they should depend absolutely. If you wish to prevent them from undertaking anything or trespassing on you it is only necessary to make them remember the *Médecin Charitable*, with which, though it only costs a sol or two, we have ruined the apothecaries of Paris. Make them understand that there are at the grocers, cassia, senna, rhubarb, syrup of roses and with these remedies we can do without them, and have rendered them so ridiculous, that no one wishes to see them at their houses, and so they have more leisure than they desire to stay in their shops. There is no more, thank God, any question of bezoar, or cordial waters in smallpox, or julep cordials, or pearls, in any disease whatever. The people are not deceived by these bagatelles or by any others. The rich do not avail themselves of them any more and hold themselves under obligation to many ancients of our Faculté for delivering them from this tyranny. These messieurs, our ancients were M. Marescot; his son-in-law, Simon Pietre; Jean Duret, son of Louis; the two Cousinots; Nicolas Pietre; Jean Hautin; M. Bouvard du Chemin; Brayer; de la Vigne; Merlet; Michel Seguin; Baralis; Alain; R. Moreau; Boujonier; Charpentier; de Launay; Guillemeau; and many others who introduced into the families at Paris an easy and familiar medical practice which has delivered them from the tyranny of these arabesque cooks.[2] . . . In such sort that the apothecaries at present scarcely find themselves in demand except for strangers lodging in furnished chambers.

[2] Figaro. Barber of Seville, Act I, Sc. iv, speaking of his functions in the house of Bartholo says he is "his barber, his surgeon, his apothecary; there is not given in his house a stroke of the razor, the lancet, or the piston except by the hand of your servant."

Writing to Spon (March 10, 1648) Patin tells him that Guillemeau had written a thesis in which he attacked the apothecaries and the Arabian pharmacy but that he had not had the courage to print it without retrenching many of the strongest parts of his arguments. Guy says "everybody is not equally brave in this country, those who think themselves wise here, worship the golden calf and revere the fortune of the wicked." Some one had said to him that "everyone was not as fortunately brave as he, and that although what he had written was right, nevertheless there was no need to say or write it." Guy pours out his contempt on such cowardice. Nevertheless one cannot help the feeling at times, that part of his bitterness, especially against the physicians who held a great place at Court, was sour grapes.

SIDE LIGHTS ON PATIN'S CLIENTELE

In a letter to Belin,[3] he says: "Most of the Court physicians are ignorant or charlatans, and very often both," and again, "at least you can go and see M. Vautier, chief physician to the King, but do not

[3] March 14, 1657.

talk to him of me; our dogs do not run together. I am not, nor do I wish to be an antimonial doctor, for I know too well that antimony is a poison." Some of those whom he judged most harshly, were certainly held in great esteem, not only by their patients but by many of their professional colleagues. Guy is not above letting his correspondents know that he has some aristocratic patients on his list. Thus he concludes a long letter to Spon (May 29, 1648): "But here is the hour that a coach should come to take me, drawn by six good horses, to see, at nine leagues from here, M. de Marillac, Master of Requests, who is sick there with an attack of gout."

The Marillacs were very prominent people and Patin liked to inform his friends of his professional relations with them. He writes to Spon (June 14, 1650) that he and the elder Moreau had been taken by the wife of M. de Marillac, *maître des requêtes*, "two leagues from here to see her sister, a nun, who was sick . . . It was beautiful in the country, and very comfortable to go there in a coach."

In a letter to Belin, *fils* (June 19, 1649) Guy says he is going against his will to Fontainbleau to see the son of a *trésorier de l'extraordinaire des guerres* who is very sick, "the father and mother take me there in their coach." The physicians of the seventeenth century made their rounds on horseback or riding a mule. There were stone steps placed at the *école de médecine* to facilitate their mounting and getting off.

Pic[4] quotes from Patin's contemporary Vigneul de Marville the following sketch of Guy which is contained in his "Mélanges d'histoire et de littérature."

Guy Patin was satiric from his head to his feet. His hat, collar, cloak, his doublet, stockings and boots, all bid defiance to the world and went to law with vanity. He had in his countenance, the air of Cicero and in his *esprit,* the character of Rabelais. His great memory furnished him always with subjects for conversation and he talked much. He was hardy, bold, inconsiderate, simple and naïve in his expressions.

In spite of some repellant characteristics Patin seems to have had a large practice chiefly among the rich bourgeoisie, the officials of the Parlement of Paris, lawyers and merchants. His professional standing was good with his colleagues in spite of his many enmities, because we know that he

[4] Guy Patin, Paris, 1911,

attended many of them, Riolan, Moreau, etc., and that he was frequently called in consultation by them.

Patin writes to Charles Spon (January 20, 1645) of a bequest of three thousand livres which he received from a patient named Jean Baptiste Lambert to whom he had been physician for eight years. Lambert had acquired a great fortune by participating in the financial affairs of the government, and Patin hints that he had given him an opportunity to join in his devious methods of acquiring wealth but adds that he had always "despised the fortune in which he wished me to share."

A sidelight on the devious ways by which some physicians sought to obtain practice in Guy's time is afforded in a letter written by him to Spon (January 7, 1661). The latter had referred a patient who was at Paris to Patin, but the patient had fallen instead into the hands of a physician named Lienard. Patin says it was probably through the agency of an inn keeper:

> Because he (Lienard) is in relation with all the hosts in his quarter and I do not doubt it if his inn was in the rue des Trois Mores or Aubry-le-Boucher, because I have known this fact for a long time . . . God be praised of all,

I do not lack patients, nor wish for them. I thank you nevertheless for your good affection. I ask you only if he is still at Lyons, without seeming to do anything, to learn from him the name of the street and sign of his inn, because I think I have divined it.

Lienard had evidently insinuated to the patient that if he fell in Patin's hands he would be bled to excess, because the patient told Spon that he had heard of this failing of Patin's. The latter says this was a cowardly trick of Lienard's similar to many others that he had done.

Patin, like other physicians, occasionally had patients stray from his fold, and he writes to Falconet (January 31, 1659) with ill-concealed despite of one such instance:

As to this Abbé Forcoal, I formerly treated him when very ill for several diseases. His father said that he wished to witness how much he thought of me and that he would give me one hundred *écus* a year to be their physician. This he did and I received this for eighteen months. The Abbé (who at that time was only *aumonier du roi*) suffered from a painful and grievous illness, from which he happily recovered and said much in praise of me. Much time passed and they did not send for me. I learned that Valot went to see them, and gave them powders, waters and pills, and that they had given me up because I prescribed too few drugs. . . . When I met the father in the city he always said he would send for me to see them, but he did not do so, so I rested there. The father was a miserable native of Cevennes, a Huguenot, who came to Paris to improve his condition, and make his fortune if he could. He was lackey to a secretary of the King's, named Addée, likewise a Huguenot, and then became his clerk. Finally, he became a great partisan and mixed in many affairs, the aides, the gabelle, and others, where he would make money. He changed his religion to become secretary to the council, and became a still greater partisan. Then he married his only daughter, who was very beautiful, to a son of M. Addée, his former master, who is blind and a Huguenot, but she was a Catholic. He had many sons, of which he made the eldest a captain, the second a *maître des requêtes*, the third *aumonier du roi*, who is now the Abbé. . . . Finally Forcoal, the father, died, owing five or six millions, with three hundred lawsuits by those whom he owed. . . .

The whole secret of these people is while they have the upper hand, to take money from all sides, and then to go into bankruptcy, not only to their creditors but likewise to God, for their conscience and their honor.

Patin gives a curious instance of his physiological views in the following statement to Falconet (October 26, 1658):

Inflammation of the lung is always fatal to those who have red hair. The late M. de la Vigne, one of the physicians of our Faculté was very red. I called him one day in consultation on a secretary of the king's named Collier who was seventy-five years old, and very redheaded. He was ill with an inflammation of the lung, which I predicted would be fatal. M. de la Vigne asked me where I had learned this prognostic of the redheaded? I answered him that I had always remarked it as very true besides which I had heard it said by M. Nicolas Pietre, who had learned it from his brother, the great Simon Pietre and the reason was that the redheaded abounded in bitter and malign serosity.

Patin certainly at times lays himself open to the reproach that those who live in glass houses should not throw stones. He retails with relish the foibles and weaknesses of his fellowmen, and consequently exposes himself to the exposure of his own. Even the dead did not escape his malicious pen. Thus he writes to Spon (January 20, 1649):

We have freshly lost one of our companions, a resolute and well-intentioned man named M. Nic Heliot, aged forty-seven years. He died of hydropsy of the lungs, after having languished for two months. He had invited in his last will, all the Faculté, as many doctors as possible to be present at his interment. To this effect he had ordained that each doctor who came there in a red robe should have two quarter crowns for his presence, and half that to those who came in a black robe with the square bonnet. He was interred with very great ceremony and pomp, accompanied by sixty doctors, of whom there were forty in red robes and twenty in black. Nevertheless the Faculté decreed that they should not take his money, and that the said sum of one hundred pounds which would have been necessary to carry out his last wishes, should be left and returned to his widow. He died without children. His brother is an *échevin* of the city of Paris. He was of a good family, very rich, but he loved extremely the ceremonies and displays that make a noise. God guard from harm those who are of an altogether different sentiment. For me I am content and much desire that they should bury me at four o'clock in the morning, or at nine o'clock in the evening, and that this *manège,* which seems only invented for the gain of priests and bell ringers, or for the solace of the living, *fiat et pereat sine sonitu,* but I hope this may not arrive too soon.

RICHELIEU AND MAZARIN

Years after Richelieu's death Patin continued to refer to him with the greatest animosity. Writing to Belin, *fils* (January 14, 1651), he speaks of a case in which a surgeon had given a narcotic pill containing opium to a patient, with a fatal result, and adds that possibly it was the same kind of pill which was given to the great Cardinal shortly before his death, which Patin thought had accelerated his end and he concludes: "Would to God he had given it to him twenty years sooner." Patin never admits that any of Richelieu's great policies were actuated by a desire to aggrandize France or the King, although it is now conceded that he was a great man who, though frequently gratifying his personal ambition, nevertheless in the main served the interests of his King and country.

His hatred of Richelieu was augmented by the fact that the Cardinal had caused the execution of de Thou, a great friend of Patin's, for treason in 1644. De Thou was the son of the famous French historian. The correspondence contains many references to the execution of young de Thou years after the event. Writing to Spon (September 12, 1664), Patin says: "It is twenty-two years ago that Armand, Cardinal de Richelieu, *Ministre enragé* had beheaded in your city my good and dear friend, M. de Thou."

There are many allusions in Patin's correspondence to Richelieu's atheism, or at least lack of belief in the fundamental doctrines of the Roman Catholic Church. Thus Patin wrote to Spon (April 13, 1657) the following anecdote:

> The Cardinal Richelieu who loved a joke when he was not tormented by his black bile, asked one day of Doctor Mulot, his confessor, how many masses were necessary to get a soul out of purgatory. Doctor Mulot responded that the Church had never defined it. The Cardinal replied: "That is because you are an ignoramus, I know very well, it requires as many of them as of bullets of snow to heat an oven." Are these not good men, who mock thus the holy and sacred fire which makes their marmite boil so fortunately?

Patin writes Spon (November 3, 1649) that a courtier had told him that two years before his death, Richelieu, notwithstanding his ill health and the immensity of his labors, had three mistresses; his niece, Marie de Vignerot, who is better known as the duchesse d'Aiguillon; Madame de Chaulnes, and the famous Marion Delorme. Of the latter Patin adds that she had been the mistress of Cinq-Mars, and many others before Richelieu: "She is still held in esteem, and has even passed into history for her beauty, because Vittorio Siri has talked of her in his 'Mercure.'"

Patin's hatred of Cardinal Mazarin, the inheritor of Richelieu's power was fully as bitter without any particular personal reason for it. One of his favorite epithets for him is "the Pantaloon in a long robe" or "the Pantaloon with a red hat." Writing to Garnier, a physician of Lyons, June 18, 1649, he says of Mazarin that it is the "Pantaloon in a long robe" who "is the cause of all our ills, and of the ruin of France."

He accuses Mazarin of finding in the wars into which he plunged France the *pierre philosophale,* and complains many times of the devastation and pillage to which the country was subjected not only by the enemies' troops but by the irregularities committed by the French troops in their own country. In a letter to Spon (May 14, 1649) he complains that his country house has been robbed by the soldiers of Mazarin, and he raises his voice many times in bitter complaints against the policies of the Cardinal. Although Mazarin's apologists point to the successful results of his diplomacy and show how the wars in which he involved France added to her territories and increased her prestige, nevertheless those who have studied the history of the period in which he controlled the destinies of the country are struck with his disregard for the sufferings of the French people and with the selfishness and avarice which dominated his actions, and must allow that there is much justice in Patin's allegations. Undoubtedly France was never in apparently greater position and prosperity than during the reign of the *Roi Soleil,* but beneath the surface of all this splendor was the misery and woe of the common people, paving the way for the events of one hundred years later. The arrogance and pride of the King of France led to the estrangement and hatred of France by other countries, and to the numerous wars from which France was to suffer throughout the eighteenth century and the ruinous financial policy which terminated in the overthrow of French royalty.

Patin's letters written during 1648–49 when the people of Paris were in revolt against the arbitrary government of Mazarin show that he sympathized with the people although he took no active part in the revolt. He retails with joy every piece of news that he picks up which would put Mazarin in a disadvantageous light. After the King, Queen Mother and the Cardinal had re-entered Paris he writes Belin, *fils*, that a printer named Morlet had been arrested for printing some scurrilous verses about the Queen Mother and Mazarin. It was a matter of current scandalous rumor that Anne of Austria and Mazarin maintained much more intimate relations than those which are customary between a regent and a chief minister of state. Patin says the printer was taken to the Châtelet and on the same day condemned to be hanged. He appealed to a higher court which confirmed the sentence. When he was being conveyed to his doom the people attacked the escort. The archers who constituted his guards fled before the savage mob, as did the executioner who rode in the cart with the prisoner. The latter escaped.

Patin tells Belin (August 27, 1649) that the Queen Mother and Mazarin were greatly afraid of what might happen to them when they returned to Paris after having had to flee from the city and then having laid seige to it: "The executioner of an Italian was so afraid for his skin." He adds that there need be no more fear of his adding any new taxes or creating new offices.

Mazarin and his agents repressed with the greatest brutality every manifestation of the sentiment of the public towards him. The animosity of the people found its chief vent in the so-called "Mazarinades," pamphlets and verses secretly printed and circulated from hand to hand in which the Cardinal was held up to ridicule and hatred in the most virulent manner. Patin writes to Spon (July 13, 1649) of a widow, named Meusnier, and her two sons who were arrested for printing some of these documents. The elder son was sentenced to be hanged, the mother was to witness the execution of her son, then to be publicly whipped, and afterwards expelled from the kingdom and the younger son was to be sent to the galleys.

When Mazarin died he left a large legacy to found the Collège des Quatre Nations, also bequeathing to France his magnificent library and the Palais Royal to the King. But this posthumous generosity did not lessen Patin's animosity. He writes Falconet (March 9, 1661):

They talk no more of the death of Mazarin. He has passed; he has folded his baggage; he is in lead the eminent personage. But they do talk of his will, of his *écus*, and they are in difficulty as to who will succeed to his political and financial all-powerfulness. They say he has left two millions to build a great college, for the instruction of poor gentlemen of four nations. One, I think, like the University at Paris or at Nevers, and that he is to be buried in the church of this college as its founder. Others say that he will be buried in Saint Denis, in France, having been its Abbé. But it little imports where they bury him, provided that he steals and tyrannizes no more over the people, as he did for too long a time. *Bon Dieu!* but their patience has been great with this tyrant. They say the college is to be built opposite the Louvre on the bank of the Seine.[5] They say that the Queen Mother is not grieved at the death of Mazarin nor is the duc d'Anjou, and that the King has quarrelled with them about it. . . . . The four nations of which I have spoken above are the Spaniards, Italians, Germans and the English. He employs the money which he has stolen in France for foreigners, not for the French.

SOCIAL LIFE IN FRANCE IN THE SEVENTEENTH CENTURY

It is very hard for the modern mind to comprehend the curious *mélange* presented

[5] It was erected there at that time. The buildings are now occupied (1920) by the Bibliothèque Mazarin and the Institute de France.

by the manners, customs, religion, superstition, erudition and ignorance, in the social life of the seventeenth century in France. Until Louis XIV attained his majority all political power was in the hands first of Richelieu, afterwards of Mazarin, both brilliant, crafty, unscrupulous ecclesiastics, who balked at no means to gratify their ambitious ends. Their rule was necessarily despotic. There yet lingered in France remains of the old feudal spirit, not yet entirely subdued to the idea of the concentration of power in the hands of a monarch. During the minorities of both Louis XIII and Louis XIV some of the great princes of France tried their best to overthrow the power held by Marie de' Médici as regent for her son, or by Anne of Austria during the minority of hers. All these attempts proved futile against the craft and ability of the two cardinals on whom the Queens successively relied, but the first half of the century is marked by a succession of treasons, stratagems and wars, only finally to end in the despotism of Louis XIV. The great Condé was for some time in arms against France, fighting with Spanish troops against his country. The social life as detailed in the memoires and letters of the time was marked by bloodshed and a looseness of morals which is almost beyond belief. Duels were so frequent and so fatal that the sternest edicts were issued against them. Every great man had a horde of parasites who would willingly commit murder or any other crime at his bidding. According to Patin even Cardinal Mazarin was guilty of having his enemies attacked by bands in his employ. He relates to Spon (November 4, 1650) that, some days before, a band of thirty armed men had attacked the coach of M. le duc de Beaufort in the rue St. Honoré. Fortunately for the latter he was not in it at the time and thus escaped the death which befell several of his servants. Patin implies that the assassins were in the employ of the Cardinal. The great nobles such as Condé, Conti, Gaston d'Orléans, all had their "men" and indulged in little private wars of their own, occasionally combining with one another against the royal authority.

The lackeys attached to the households of the nobles were a great source of trouble. They adopted the insolent bearing and manners of their masters and were involved in continual broils among themselves or with the citizens. Patin in a letter to Falconet (January 26, 1655) relates a typical incident:

A young gentleman, a captain of the guards, named M. de Tilladet, whose father yet living was once governor of Bapaume and later of Brissac, nephew of M. le Tellier, secretary of state, was miserably killed by the pages and lackeys of M. d'Espernon. The carrosses of the two masters met and ran into one another. The lackeys tried to kill the coachman of M. de Tilladet. The master jumped from his coach to prevent them, was overwhelmed by these rascals and brutally killed. The King wishes justice should be done and has issued a proclamation against lackeys in order to prevent such abuses, to wit that they shall not carry swords or firearms in the future, on pain of death; and they shall henceforth dress in suits of various colors, and not in gray, in order that they may be recognized. This proclamation was sent to Parlement to be certified and published. This has been done. It is affixed on all the squares and published throughout the city, but I do not know for how long a time it will be observed. The Jesuits say that the decrees of the Sorbonne last no longer than a week. Perhaps it will be the same with these ordinances, because the French people make many good regulations but observe them badly.

Many of the great ladies of the court indulged in the most shameless intrigues. Mazarin was accused of being the lover of Marie de' Médici, and by many of being the father of Louis XIV. Marguerite de Valois and the duchesse de Navarre are said to have had the heads of their respective lovers, Coconas and La Mole embalmed after they had been beheaded for treason and to have kept these gruesome relics as trophies of their affection. The court was full of bastards of high lineage for whom provision was made at the public expense by the gift of political or ecclesiastical benefices.

Murders were so frequent among the nobility that they only excited momentary interest. The wicked and eccentric Queen Christina of Sweden after her abdication while staying at Fontainebleau caused one of her household named Monaldeschi to be murdered in the hall of the palace. For a short time the court was horrified but a few weeks later she was in Paris, fêted and entertained as if nothing had happened.

Although there are frequent references in the "Letters" to the famous blue-stocking Queen, Christina of Sweden, Patin seems never to have met her personally. Writing to Falconet (October 6, 1656) he says:

The Queen of Sweden has not been in Paris as much as she had wished. She has seen next to nothing of it. Nevertheless she has received the approbation of all those who have met her here. She has much presence of mind and perception. She is neither stupid nor bigoted. She loves neither women nor girls. She understands Latin well and knows more of it than many men who profess to do so. I know from a good source that when twenty-three years old she knew all Martial by heart. They say she makes much of Catullus, the tragedies of Seneca, and yet more of Lucian. . . . As to her conversion, brought about by the Jesuits, I do not know what to say of it. My deceased father told me that the fat M. du Maine (Mayenne) chief of the League, said that princes had no religion until they had passed the age of forty when they became old and wise, or at least should become so. When I consider the course of this Queen during the past two years, I recall the story of a certain Italian, who suffered from *pérégrinomanie,* or the mania for traveling. He came to Geneva and after having seen how the ministers lived, was asked by them what he thought of their religion. "It is not so bad," he replied, "but ours is more useful in traveling." Thus, in the design which she has to travel in different countries, she can well take the advice of this Italian, and beyond doubt she could not easily see Rome, the Pope, and the many butterflies that are there, without travesting herself as she has done, whether she has done it seriously or not.

The Marquis de Charton was murdered as he came out from mass at the church of the Augustines. Patin tells with some gusto how one of his murderers was beheaded and the other broken on the wheel.

ABORTION

Abortion was an antisocial crime which prevailed to a terrible extent in the highest social circles in France during the seventeenth century. Bayle[6] devotes one of his most interesting marginalia to a discussion of the question. In spite of civil and ecclesiastical decrees and proclamations and of the special abhorrence with which the crime was regarded by the Church of Rome, the *grandes dames* of the time made light of the earthly and spiritual terrors which were held up to them and persistently resorted to crime to conceal their shame. Bayle uses this to support the thesis that the fear of

[6] Dictionnaire biographique. Guy Patin.

worldly shame is a stronger sentiment than that of religion. There was a large class of men and women who practiced abortion as a specialty, the latter drawn chiefly from the ranks of the midwives. It was estimated that over six hundred cases were known to have occurred, the greater part among women of high social position, in less than one year in Paris alone. Patin writes to Falconet (June 22, 1660) of a very notorious case of this kind; Mademoiselle de Guerchi had been seduced by the duc de Vitry:

They make a great clamor here about the death of Mademoiselle de Guerchi. They had imprisoned the midwife at the Châtelet, but she has been taken from there to the conciergerie by order of the Court. The curé of Saint Eustache has refused sepulture to the body of the lady. They say that it was carried to the hotel de Condé, and was there put in quicklime in order to consume it soon, so that it could not be identified if anyone came to see it. The midwife has defended herself well up to now. . . . But I believe the question will be put to her. The vicars-general and the plenipotentiaries went to complain to the Premier President that in a year six hundred women, by actual count, have confessed to killing and destroying their fruit.

The midwife of Mademoiselle de Guerchi, a woman named Constantin admitted that the lady had died in her house but denied having given her any abortifacient. She said she was told that the patient had taken some medicine, but that when she first saw her she was so very ill that there was nothing to do but to try to alleviate her sufferings. The Premier President and the *lieutenant criminel* consulted Patin about the case. A surgeon, named Le Large, was accused of complicity, but managed to exculpate himself though Patin thought his excuses very lame. The midwife was found guilty and hung at the Croix du Trahoir, as Guy says *en belle companie.*

The midwives were under regulation in the sixteenth century, and their moral character as well as their professional qualifications were looked into very carefully. Patin writes to Falconet (September 14, 1660) that he had been appointed by the Premier President to hold an examination for the appointment of a midwife to the Hôtel-Dieu, not only to serve the patients there but also to teach her profession in its wards. Thus the vast clinical material in the enormous hospital was utilized for teaching purposes at a time when clinical teaching was almost unknown elsewhere. Blondel, the Dean of the Faculté de Médecine, officiated with Patin at the examination, and a short time afterwards they held another examination for the purpose of choosing a lithotomist to the Hôtel-Dieu.

The clergy were as depraved as their flocks. Their charges were openly bought and sold, and those who had enough money and influence would accumulate a number of benefices which they shamelessly neglected except for the collection of the incomes due from them. The lives of many of the most prominent ecclesiastics were shockingly immoral and fully justify the many aspersions which Patin casts upon what he sarcastically terms the sacred institution of celibacy. The Jesuits though not so openly immoral in their lives were ambitious and constantly mingling in political affairs. The one bright spot in the religious life of the time was afforded by the followers of Jansen, the Port Royalists, and they were looked upon with suspicion and hatred by the authorities of the Roman Catholic Church because of their alleged heterodoxy but especially because of their open reprobation of the disorderly lives of their fellow clergy and the earnest efforts which they made to purify the church. To the non-medical student of the times, Patin's letters are full of interest because of their constant references to current events and to the great personages who figured in them.

LOUIS XIV AND MEDICINE

Garrison[7] directs attention to three episodes in the life of Louis XIV which had a great effect on the medical profession in France. In 1657 the King had an attack of what was probably typhoid fever. His recovery was attributed by many to the antimony which was administered to him by his physicians. The result was a great increase in the vogue of antimony, so much so that a few years later it was restored to the official pharmacopœia. It is needless to say that Patin did not agree in this opinion. In his correspondence he refers in a number of letters to the King's illness. He had been taken ill while with the army and was conveyed from the camp in Flanders to Calais. From contemporary accounts there is but little doubt that his illness was typhoid fever, although, of course, that name was not given to it at that

[7] Garrison, F. History of medicine, Introduction. Philadelphia, 1921.

time. He was very sick and consternation prevailed throughout France. Prayers were offered in all the churches, and Valot, Guénault and Daquin were in constant attendance at his bedside. "Here is a powerful King of France in good hands! Would you not say that charlatans are only suffered and tolerated to maltreat princes!" The King recovered, and Patin writes Spon that he has received an account of his illness from one who was with him:

I assure you that the King took only one third of an ounce of *vin émétique,* because the ounce had been put in three ounces of infusion of cassia and senna, and inasmuch as the first dose operated too much, he did not take the two others, but it was necessary to bleed him, finding him much worse and he has also been bled many times since. So that the King does not owe his recovery at all to this deathbearing (*mortifere*) remedy. If the King had died one would never cease to reproach them for having poisoned him, and they put themselves in great danger of such a reproach.

In spite of Patin's judgment the great majority of his subjects attributed the King's recovery to the "antimonialists" and thought that their sovereign remedy was the chief factor in the happy result.

The case certainly redounded to their credit and greatly increased their reputation.

With the other two medical episodes in the reign of Louis XIV, Patin's correspondence has no connection, but they are of so much interest that I will briefly mention them. In 1663 when the mistress of Louis XIV, Louise de la Vallière, was confined she was attended by Boucher, a man. This had an immense influence in furthering the cause of male midwifery. It is said that Louis XIV watched the proceedings from the concealment of some curtains. In 1686 the King suffered from an anal fistula of which he was cured by an operation performed by the surgeon, Félix. The happy result brought about an immediate change in the status of the French surgeons as the King interested himself in improving it. It may be recalled as an instance of courtly servility that many of the courtiers, although not suffering from any trouble of a similar nature insisted on submitting themselves to a like operation in order to show their submissive devotion to their royal master, and that those who had not sufficient nerve actually to subject themselves to the dangers and discomforts of an operation pretended to have done so and had dressings ostentatiously applied to their anal region in order to deceive the public.

Patin was a great admirer of Louis XIV and in a letter to Falconet (August 26, 1667) he tells him with satisfaction that the King realizing that many officers and men in his army then campaigning in Flanders lost their lives from lack of medical care, had sent to Paris for three surgeons to serve with the army. A physician was also to accompany them to act as chief of the medical service and to govern the hospital. It should be recalled that at this epoch there was no organized medical service with the armies. The kings or great nobles who went to war were accompanied by surgeons just as in the time of Ambroise Paré.

PARIS AND THE COURT

Patin was born in 1601, he was therefore a boy of eight when Henri IV was assassinated by the monk, Ravaillac, at the instigation of the Jesuits, and his hatred of the monks and Jesuits can be traced to the early remembrance of the horror with which the right-thinking people of France were inspired by it, and to the early influence of the terror under which the Leaguers held

France during the last quarter of the sixteenth century. He came to Paris as a young man and lived there until his death in 1672, never leaving the city except for a few very short journeys. Although not one of those courtly physicians who held lucrative positions at Court about the person of the King or some of the great nobles, the "Letters" gives glimpses of the ailments from which these grand people suffered. In them he retails much gossip of their doings and reflects the current opinions about them. The death of Richelieu, closely followed by that of Louis XIII in 1643, was a matter of vital interest to so zealous a guardian of the privileges of the Faculté de Médecine, and the great hopes which centered on Louis XIV, were shared by him in common with all Frenchmen of the time. The disorders incident to the Fronde, that very disturbing family quarrel, figure at length in his pages, interspersed with dissertations on the newest books, or recent acquisitions of fine editions of old ones for his library. We would not expect, nor do we find him taking any active part in the stirring events which kept Paris in a turmoil throughout his life. He writes of them as an interested spectator, manifesting considerable partisanship in the expression of his views but not precipitating himself into the vortex. The longest letter of Patin which we possess is one written to Spon, bearing dates on different days throughout January, February and March, 1649, in which he relates the events in the warfare between the Parlement of Paris, and the party of the Queen Mother and Mazarin, whom he hated as much as he had his predecessor, Richelieu. He writes with the greatest freedom of all the great personages who were mixed in it, and particularly emphasizes the love of the Queen Mother, Anne of Austria, for the Cardinal. To the student of this epoch this letter is invaluable for its vivid word pictures and the excellent summary it presents of the views of the people of Paris, and their Parlement in their memorable effort to overthrow the tyranny of the Cardinal and his royal mistress. It will be remembered that the Queen Mother acting as regent for her son, Louis XIV, then a mere boy had ordered the arrest of Blancmesnil and Broussel, two of the most respected members of the Parlement, and especially respected for the stand they took in opposition to Mazarin. At the news of their arrest the citizens rose *en masse:* The

Queen Mother, the young King, and Mazarin fled to St. Germain, and surrounding the city with troops tried to reduce the rebellious populace to their authority. The Royal party patched up a reconciliation between themselves and their former declared enemy, the prince de Condé, and he was given command of the royal troops. The prince de Conti, Elboeuf and de Longueville were the chief leaders of the people's party.

One of the noblemen who took the part of the Parisians in their struggle against the despotism of Mazarin was the duc de Beaufort, son of the duc de Vendôme. The *Dames des Halles,* or marketwomen of Paris, played a prominent part in many of the political disturbances in that city, and during the Fronde they made themselves conspicuous on the popular side. Patin writes Spon (May 14, 1649) the following curious particulars about the young Duke and his female admirers:

They talk of nothing here but of M. le duc de Beaufort, for whom the Parisians, and particularly all the women, have a very special devotion. As he was playing tennis in a resort in the Marais du Temple, four days ago, most of the women of the Halles (markets) went by platoons to see him play and offered vows for his prosperity. As they made a great tumult to get in and those in the place complained about it, it was necessary for him to quit playing and come to the door to put them off. This he could not do without permitting a small number of the women to enter, one after the other, to see him play. Seeing that one of the women regarded him with amiability he said to her: "Eh, my gossip, you wanted to come in. What pleasure do you get in watching me play and seeing me lose my money?" She answered him at once, "Monsieur de Beaufort play hardily, you will not want for money, my *commère* who is here with me and I, have brought you two hundred *écus*, and if more is needed, I am ready to go back and seek as much again." All the other women commenced to cry also that their money was at his service, for which he thanked them. He was visited that day by more than two thousand women. Two days later, passing by Saint Eustache, a troop of women commenced to cry to him: "Monsieur, do not consent to marry the niece of Mazarin, whatever M. de Vendôme does or says to you. If he abandons you, you will lack nothing. We will give you a pension every year of sixty thousand livres in the Halles." He has proclaimed that if they persecute him at Court, in order to be in safe keeping he would lodge in the center of the markets, where more than twenty thousand women would guard him. This event caused more amusement than fear, but here is worse. This prince, aged thirty-two years, having overheated himself, drank of wine and beer, and suffered much pain in the kidneys, during which time he also vomited many times. When this was known in Paris, the people believed he had been poisoned at Mazarin's order. His house was soon filled with an infinity of men and women. Even M. de Vendôme, his father, who is here now, believed he had been poisoned, and when the physicians assured him that he had not, he warned them that the poison was Italian, and that the Italians were subtler poisoners than the French. But at length he is cured and the Italians are cleared of that of which they were suspected.

The people suspected, not without reason, that many of the nobility who acted as their partisans and by virtue of their rank and military experience commanded them in their conflict with the regular troops also served the Queen Mother and Mazarin. De Longueville left Paris on an expedition into Normandy to raise troops and to procure provisions. He left with the Parisians, as hostages, his wife and eldest son. Patin tells how during his absence Madame de Longueville gave birth to another son, who was appropriately christened Charles Paris de Longueville, comte de Saint Paul, his godparents being the provost of the merchants, the president of the Parlement, and four aldermen of the city of Paris. The baby grew up and Madame de Sévigné describes his death in 1672, when he was killed on the banks of the Rhine as Louis XIV's army was entering Germany.

The mistrust of the people was justified by the discovery that a number of persons of high position who had remained in Paris were acting as spies and conveying information to the Mazarinists, as those who surrounded the young King were termed by the Frondeurs. Apropos of these spies Patin writes to Spon (February 20, 1649): "All these miserable hangdogs, men of quality and dignity make themselves spies for a foreigner, a trickster, a comedian; sell and betray their country and take the part of an Italian who is only good to be chased from it." Patin says that if Mazarin was compelled to flee from France he would not be able to go to Rome because the Pope was Pamphilio, and Mazarin had caused the murder of a nephew of the latter's, which the uncle would promptly avenge. If he fled to Venice, where he was said to have accumulated money and goods in preparation for a rainy day, the Pope would deprive him of his cardinalate and perhaps have him assassinated. Patin says that those who know him well think he would do better to go to Turkey, have himself circumcised, and trust to the mercy of the Grand Turk and his mufti rather than to that of the Pope, Cardinal Pamphilio, or Cardinal Panciról, another prelate who had great influence with the Pope and was an avowed enemy of Mazarin. Later when the Court was at Saint Germain because of the rebellious attitude of the people, Patin says that many would like to march on Saint Germain, bring the King and his Mother back to Paris, and execute the Cardinal on the Place de la Grève:

> This to be done as an example to posterity, and to teach Italians not to come here and place themselves so easily at Court, to the desolation and total ruin of a flourishing kingdom, as the Marquis d'Ancre wished to do in other times, but together with his wife and his followers in the end had made a bad bargain of it. Please God for the welfare of France that it was likewise with Mazarin. Helas! but we would be fortunate.

The so-called war was conducted with but little spirit by the military leaders on either side. The great Turenne lent his support to the Parlement side but took no very great part in the affair. There were many skirmishes but no real battles, and food seems to have been brought into Paris in sufficient quantities to prevent any real distress. Patin writes that he has "thank God! flour, bread, and wheat sufficient for more than a month for me and my family, with wine, money, and provisions for a much longer time, and though I am in a blockaded city, half besieged, I have no need nor want." Finally a peace was concluded, which although it gave temporary satisfaction to the people yielded them no permanent advantages. Patin's letter intermixes with his account of these events much bibliographic gossip and medical news.

Patin describes to Spon (August 20, 1649) most graphically the return of the Court to Paris, and the reconciliation that ensued:

Finally the Queen Mother has returned to Paris bringing with her the King, at the solicitation of the two princes of the blood (duc d'Anjou and the duc d'Orléans), although she had no desire to do so, and Mazarin even less. He (the King) arrived here Friday, the 18th of this month, at eight o'clock in the evening, in a great coach which was very full. Among those with him in it were M. le duc d'Anjou, M. le duc d'Orléans, M. le prince de Condé, and Mazarin, who was so ashamed that he hid himself so that one could scarcely see him. There were also the Queen Mother, Madame la duchesse d'Orléans, Mademoiselle, and Madame, la princesse de Condé, *la douairière,* and the maréchal de Villeroi. Many of the city companies marched in advance. They entered by the rue Saint-Denis, went the length of the street until beyond the (Fountain of the) Innocents, then entered the rue de la Ferronnerie (in which the late King Henri IV was killed), and passing the entire length of the rue Saint Honoré entered into the Palais Cardinal, and all this journey was made among so many acclamations and so much joy of the people that there could not have been more. I, who am talking to you, who naturally hate ceremonies, seeing the great commotion that there was in the city, and the joy of everybody in it, was there also, and saw more kinds of people in greater numbers than I ever saw before. The Queen Mother said in the evening, while supping at the Palais Cardinal, that she had never believed that the people of Paris had loved the King so much.

Patin took but little delight in the gorgeous spectacles in which the inhabitants of Paris have from time immemorial taken so great a pleasure. Writing to Spon[8] he tells him of the entry into Paris of the ambassadors of Poland who were sent to ask the Princess Marie to become their Queen:

The entry was made with such pomp as one has never seen the like. They entered by the Porte Saint Honoré to the Hôtel de Vendôme, so that they had passed across Paris from end to end, also they were seen by an infinite number of people who ran in the morning to hold their place on the streets whereby they would pass. All that day I was very busy with people who had not strength to quit their beds, but I assure you that in the other streets where they did not pass, there was so great a solitude, that it seemed to me like a city deserted by famine or pestilence, from which I pray God he will preserve you and me. I could have gone out to the Porte Saint Antoine, where I could have seen everything easily, but I did not wish to take the trouble. These public spectacles scarcely touch me, they render me melancholy. I, who am naturally joyous and gay, instead of rejoicing in them as others do, when I see all this crowd, pity the vanity of those who cause it. It is true that these shows are not made for philosophers of the humor and capacity of which I would wish to be, but they are for the vulgar who are dazzled by this *éclat* and pass the time more pleas-

[2] November 16, 1645.

antly because of it. That day I was longer than usual in my study and employed myself there sufficiently well. My neighbors said I did very wrong in not having been at the ceremony, and that it was the most beautiful thing in the world. They reproach me that I have too little curiosity and too much melancholy, and I say they are too wasteful of their time. I appeal to you about it. If you condemn me I promise you that the first time the Pope will come to Paris, I will go expressly to the rue Saint-Jacques ahead of him, where I will await him in a bookseller's in reading some books, and it will be only to please you, because if King Solomon with the Queen of Sheba made their entrée in all their glory, I know not if I would quit my books for them. My study pleases me far otherwise, and I keep myself there more willingly than in the most beautiful palace of Paris.

When Christina, Queen of Sweden, made her visit to Paris in September, 1656, Patin seems to have departed from his usual custom for he writes to Charles Spon (September 13, 1656):

The Queen of Sweden has made her entrée into Paris, where she has been received with great magnificence. She entered by torchlight. It was nine o'clock in the evening when she passed over the Pont Notre-Dame. I never saw so many people as there were in the streets when she passed. She was on horseback, immediately behind a beautiful dais that they carried before her. She had on a red jacket, a *perruque*, and a hat over her ear.

Perhaps Patin condescended to witness her entrance because of her patronage of learning.

Patin's correspondence in 1660 is full of the joy which was felt throughout France at the marriage of Louis XIV with the Infanta of Spain. It was believed that thereby the long and wearisome wars, both civil and foreign, in which the country had been almost continuously engaged since the death of Henri IV would be terminated. Nevertheless Patin growls at the tumult which agitated Paris on the occasion of the entry into the capital of the young King with his bride. Guy even meditated a temporary sojourn away from his beloved city. He writes Falconet (August 20, 1660):

We have here nothing but the noise of drums, and of soldiers, and I believe, until the fête is over we shall not have better times. I have some Latin to do, which is commenced but cannot be finished in this noise. I would be at Lyons with you for a week; we could converse together, *inter privatos parietes*, of many things *quae litteris non consignantur*, and after the tumult had lessened here, I would return by Roanne to Orleans by the Loire. . . . Our profession makes slaves of us. I shall never have any repose until I shall be buried and then they can make an epitaph for me similar to that of the Maréchal of France, named Trivulce, a Milanese, who lies buried in the Church of Saint-Nazaire at Milan, *hic quiescit qui numquam quievit* (here rests one who until now never rested). I have menaced my son, Charles, with it, who is always studying and never rests.

Five days later Patin writes Falconet that he had been one of those who officially represented the University of Paris at the formal entry of the King and his bride. The various faculties assembled at five o'clock in the morning at the Church of the Mathurins in their official robes and headed by the rector, who had to deliver a formal address to the King, marched to the place assigned to them in the faubourg Saint-Antoine. "There were thirty-eight doctors of medicine in their red robes, who were much gazed at," says Patin with evident pride.

Even an ordinary journey of the court must have constituted a wonderful spectacle. Patin[9] records that when Louis XIV went to Dijon the royal party traveled in

[9] Letter to Falconet, October 25, 1658.

one hundred and ten carrosses each drawn by six horses, besides which there were the saddle horses and those which carried the luggage.

Anne of Austria, mother of Louis XIV, died of a cancer of the breast on January 20, 1666. She had been ill for a long time and Patin's letters contain many references to the various charlatans who were called in to try their remedies on her during the last year of her life. In spite of the fact that she manifested friendship for Mazarin, Patin speaks with admiration of her management of affairs during the minority of her son. Readers of Dumas will find interesting the references made by Patin to the trial and disgrace of Fouquet, and to many of the other characters who figure in the immortal pages of that writer of romance.

Patin sympathized with Fouquet. In his Letters written during the period of his trial he retails much information throwing light on the sentiments of his contemporaries. Fouquet was tried before twenty-two judges, nine of whom voted for his death, the balance for perpetual banishment. Patin thought the King wished him to receive the death penalty. Be that as it may, the sentence was finally changed into imprisonment for life. In 1664 he was sent to Pignerol, where he was closely confined until his death in 1680. At the trial of the Maréchal de Marillac in 1632, Fouquet was the only one of his judges who was brave enough to withstand the desires of Richelieu and vote against the infliction of the death penalty. He thus incurred the great Cardinal's displeasure and only received the highest charges of the state during the regime of Mazarin. It is interesting that when he was himself in peril of his life he also was fortunate in finding those who bravely withstood the wishes of Louis XIV. His chief defenders at the trial were d'Ormesson and de Roquesant. Patin hints in a letter to Falconet (December 21, 1664) that Fouquet might be poisoned in his prison:

When one is within four walls one does not eat what he wishes or sometimes eats more than he wishes; and, moreover Pignerol produces truffles and mushrooms. Sometimes they mix with them sauces which are dangerous for us French, when they are served by Italians. That which is good is that the King has never caused anyone to be poisoned, and has an upright and generous soul, but can one say as much for those who govern under his authority.

Monsieur de la Roquesant was exiled into Brittany because of his brave defense of Fouquet. He was allowed to return to Paris in 1667, and Patin showed his appreciation of his honorable behavior by refusing to take a fee when called in to attend him.

Patin writes to Falconet (June 22, 1660) the following amusing account of a little trip that he and his wife made to Saint-Denis with his son, Robert, and his bride:

Will you pardon me, Monsieur, if I write you of the debauch I made today, Tuesday, June 22nd? I let myself be taken by my wife and our two newly wedded ones to Saint-Denis, where I saw the fair, which was a poor thing. The church is beautiful but a little dark. In the treasury there are many toys and foolish things, *pro more gentis*. At the tombs of the kings I could not refrain from weeping, seeing so many monuments of the vanity of human life. Some tears escaped me, likewise, at the grave of the great and good King François I, who founded our Royal College. It is necessary that I confess to you my weakness, I even kissed it and that of his father-in-law Louis XII, who was the father of his people and the best king we ever had in France. There are no tombs erected as yet for the Bourbons. . . .

In the choir, on the right hand, beneath the grand altar, they have put during the last few days the duc d'Orléans, who died at Blois, February 2nd, on the seventh day of a continued fever, with a fluxion of the chest and four doses of *vin émétique*, of which Guénault ordered the three last, saying it was the true method of curing him. . . . My wife was ravished with these bagatelles, and took for so many truths the little tales which were told her by a monk authorizing them with his wand. I was already informed of these foolishnesses when I was at Saint-Denis at the funeral of King Louis XIII, with our Dean, M. de la Vigne, in 1642.

PUBLIC EXECUTIONS

Although Patin does not seem to have been possessed by the same morbid desires which led Charles Selwyn to attend, on every possible occasion, the executions of criminals; he nevertheless seems to have had a keen relish for the details of such events, and in his letters we find descriptions of terrible crimes and often much more terrible punishments interspersed with grave dissertations on professional topics or tranquil recitals of bibliographic data. Pic, though not attempting any explanation, points out that mention of executions and crimes are comparatively rare in Patin's correspondence until the year 1654 from which time they increase *ad nauseam.*

Thus he writes to Spon, on repeated occasions of the murder of a *valet de chambre* in the house of the duc d'Orléans in Paris, and of the subsequent execution of two men and a woman for the crime. The woman was hanged but the two men were broken alive on the wheel and old Guy recites with vivacity their sufferings before death kindly terminated them. On one occasion he writes of an execution which must have given him a thrill of exultation:

> At five o'clock yesterday, at the gate of Paris, they hung a chemist (who called himself a Provençal gentleman) for forgery. He was from Avignon. He said he prepared his antimony in furnaces where he made the false money. He was caught in the act and has been hanged from the end of a beam.

The joy at seeing an antimonialist being hung for counterfeiting must have been great to Guy.

He writes Spon (May 19, 1648) that "on that day they had broken on the wheel two highwaymen, one of whom confessed that he killed more than thirty men."

Patin was filled with an unholy joy whenever an ecclesiastic was found guilty of any criminality and his letters contain many references to such cases, accompanied by comments such as he writes in telling Belin, *fils* (May 7, 1660) of a priest who was hanged and burned on the preceding Tuesday, "who was a bad rascal . . . There are two others yet in the Châtelet who are no better . . . The holy and sacred celibacy of priests fills the world with prostitutes, cuckolds, and bastards."

There was a Breton priest, Jean Cricant, whose execution Patin in a letter to Charles Spon (September 19, 1657) relates with some exultation. This man had been secretary and almoner to the bishop of Auxerre, but had seduced a nun and brought her to Paris, where he lived with her and gained a scanty living by practicing quackery. Patin had a patient with epilepsy to whom he had told the truth, that his case was incurable. The ex-priest promised to cure him by means of certain pills. The remedy made the poor patient worse and he brought suit against the quack to recover the money he had paid him. He laid bare the evil life of the man, and consequently the quack and the nun were brought to trial for their immorality. The man was hanged and burned at the Gréve, and the nun was sent to the Madelonnettes.

On August 4, 1670, a young man, named Pierre Sarrazin, attacked with a sword a priest who was saying mass at Notre-Dame, wounding him in two places. A few days later Patin writes about the affair to Falconet. He says he was a Huguenot of Caen, and that he believes him to have been out of his mind. Sarrazin was tried at once and on the very next day was burnt at the Gréve, after having first been paraded in front of Notre-Dame. Patin says he gave vent to no expressions of piety or religion, nor of regret at dying.

To Falconet he writes (June 16, 1650) of a robbery and murder committed by a band of men of whom five had been captured and broken on the wheel, two were yet in prison, and nine had escaped:

I am much vexed that they have not the nine others, in order that they should undergo the punishment they merit. Is not the devil unchained in Christendom that such crimes are committed by such men in the center of Paris? Do they do worse in Turkey, where they do not preach the Evangel of the Messiah, and where there are no monks? As for me, I believe the end of the world will come soon when I see so many iniquities.

He tells Spon (January 11, 1655): "They have just broken alive at the Croix du Trahoir a wicked hangdog and great thief named Delussel, *enfant de Paris*, aged twenty-eight years. I have never seen so many people gathered on the streets of Paris as there were to see him pass."

Nevertheless, to judge from the following, Patin did not like the sickening sights which were presented by the prisons of those days. He writes to Spon (April 24, 1657) that a young man had been tried for a theft at the Châtelet, and sentenced to be hanged. When the sentence was pronounced he fell in an apoplexy. "Messieurs du Châtelet asked me to go and see him, but I could not decide to do it, the prison horrifies me so much. I was once sickened for three months by it and have not the heart to return there."

Writing to Belin, *fils* (October 8, 1655) Patin tells him that during that week he had made a public dissection, before a large audience, of a woman twenty-five years old who had been executed for counterfeiting.

During the seventeenth century in France there was a great deal of discussion of the subject of demoniacal possession, a subject upon which Guy writes with great *éclat* and with a remarkable modernity of judgment and spirit. At the beginning of the century Martha Brossier, had succeeded in achieving great notoriety, pretending to be possessed by a demon and to have the power of exorcism. She seems to have been a nervous, hysterical young woman who traveled about France with her father using her psychopathy as a means of procuring a livelihood. She finally came to Paris and displayed her occult phenomena, particularly at the Church of Sainte Geneviève. The Bishop of Paris appointed a commission of physicians to examine her, and they reported that she was a neurasthenic and a fraud, and that they could find no evidence of any supernatural agency in her acts. The Parlement of Paris finally ordered her imprisoned. She was released and taken to Rome by a couple of ecclesiastics who hoped to exploit her for their benefit on that particularly favorable soil, but the cardinal d'Ossat, having heard of her previous career cut short their project by causing her to be imprisoned in a convent. Simon Pietre wrote a treatise on the Brossier woman which he published under the name of Michel Marescot in which he showed the falsity of her claims.

Another famous case of supposed demoniac possession was that of Urbain Grandier, curé of the Church of St. Peter at Loudun, executed in 1634 as a sorcerer, and in support of whose claim to supernatural powers many books were written. Guy, in a letter to Spon (November 16, 1643), says that his execution was brought about by the malice of Cardinal Richelieu, concerning whom Grandier had published a libellous pamphlet.

Patin[10] relates the end of the son of Laubardemont, the *maitre des requêtes* who presided at the trial of Grandier:

> The ninth of this month, at nine in the evening, a carosse was attacked by robbers. The noise caused the citizens to run forth from their houses, as much perhaps from curiosity as from charity. There was firing on one part and on the other.

[10] Letter to Falconet, December 22, 1651.

One of the robbers was stretched on the pavement and a lackey of theirs arrested, the rest ran away. The wounded man died the next morning without making any statement, not complaining or stating who he was. At last he was identified. They know that he was the son of the *maitre des requêtes*, named Laubardemont, who condemned to death in 1639 the poor curé Urbain Grandier, and had him burned alive, under the charge of having sent the devil into the society of the nuns of Loudun, whom they taught to dance in order to persuade the foolish that they were possessed by the devil. Is not this a divine punishment in the family of this unfortunate judge, to expiate, in some sort the cruel death of that poor priest, whose blood cries for vengeance.

Readers of Alfred de Vigny's celebrated romance "Cinq Mars" will recall the very different ending of Laubardemont's son in that book. Otherwise de Vigny's story of the Grandier affair is very close to the facts as we know them, with the exception of the insanity of the nun, which is not recorded in history. Patin had a friend who was closely concerned in the scandal, namely, Claude Quillet, who was one of the curious characters of the time. After practicing medicine with considerable success he became a priest.

Born at Chinon in 1602 he died at Paris in 1661. He was summoned to Loudun at the time of the outbreak of hysteria among the nuns to assist at their examination. Later when some of the nuns at Chinon attempted a somewhat similar hysterical manifestation Quillet wrote some satirical verses in Latin about them. These offended Cardinal Mazarin and Quillet found it wise to join the suite of the Marechal d'Estrees, the French ambassador at Rome, and remain for a time in voluntary exile.

While at Rome Quillet composed his famous poem "Callipaedia, or the Art of making Beautiful Children," which was published at Leiden in 1655. It enjoyed great popularity and was translated into French and English.

Patin says he often talked with him and found him both witty and wise.

Patin in a letter to Charles Spon (June 14, 1657) tells of visiting a patient one evening at whose house he found a choice gathering of wits and literary men, including M. de Montmaur, Marolles, Sorel, the author of Françion and of the Berger Extravagant, and the Abbé Quillet. He says that many good things were said, "about the pope, cardinals, and monks" and he sends Spon a copy of a verse which one of the company retailed:

O la belle fiction,
O la rare invection
Que ce feu du purgatoire!
Le pape n'était pas sot,
Qui nous donna cette histoire
Pour faire bouillir son pot.

They had a mutual friend in Gassendi, at whose house they must have frequently encountered one another. Patin says the Abbé (he was usually known by his ecclesiastical, not his medical title) was "a great red fellow with a short neck."

In de Vigny's novel the Abbé Quillet figures as the hero's tutor. He is represented as actually taking the part of Urbain Grandier.

Patin states that in all these *possessions modernes* those concerned are always women or girls, bigots or nuns, priests or monks, and that it is not a devil of hell that is responsible for them but a devil of the flesh, engendered by the holy and sacred celibacy, or it is rather hysteromania than a true demonomania. He accuses the monks of having favored such demonstrations in order to increase the demand for holy water, otherwise greatly diminished by the writings of Luther and Calvin. He adds as proof that one sees no such cases in Holland, Germany or England, where there are but few monks and priests. The best of all writings on the subject he thinks is the book by Johan W. Weyer, John Wier or Joannes Wierus, "De praestigiis daemonum," but Guy gives a long sort of *catalogue raisonné* of books on the subject, by which it is plain to see he had devoted considerable time to the study of the literature of the matter. He refers among others to the writings of Bodineau, Caesalpinus, Charpentier or Carpentarius, Duncan, Riolan and Pietre. He adds:

A certain Thyrocus, a German loyolite (Jesuit) has written much on this business, but there is nothing of value in all that he has written. You would say that these master monks had assumed the task of making known the devil, and showing his claws to the world, in order that one would have recourse to their spiritual toys and holy grains.

It is curious to compare the views of Patin on the subject of witchcraft with those of his English contemporary, Sir Thomas Browne.

Besides the works of Sir Thomas Browne, Patin was familiar with those of other

English authors. Writing to Belin, *fils*, (October 28, 1658) he says: "Bacon was a chancellor of England who died in 1626, and was a great personage, a mind curious and elevated. All that he wrote is good."

Saumaise, the literary antagonist of Milton, was a friend of Patin's who refers to his book against Milton. Patin speaks of him as *l'excellent et l'incomparable personage.*

In one of his letters[11] Patin excites our curiosity by telling Spon of a wonderful invention by an Englishman, the son of a Frenchman, which is able to run a coach from Paris to Fontainebleau, "without horses by wonderful springs. They say this new machine is being prepared in the Temple. If the design succeeds it will save much hay and oats, which are of an extreme dearness."

LAST DAYS

Concerning the last years of Guy Patin's life we have but little information. After the Faculté de Médecine, March, 1660, had solemnly declared its approval of antimony, Patin seems to have lost his interest in its affairs, or at least to have retired from active participation in them. Of one hundred and

[11] To Spon, January 20, 1645.

two of its members, ninety-two had voted in favor of the repeal of the decree against it. It must have been a bitter blow to the old man when the institution, of whose fame and interests he had been such a zealous partizan, declared itself so decisively in opposition to his cherished prejudice. He continued his correspondence with his friends in Lyons but the tone of the letters is even more embittered than in earlier years, and the depression of his spirits is marked. The death of his eldest son, the exile of Charles, and the triumph of his professional rivals all depressed and worried his advancing years. The last letter of Patin in the collection published by Reveillé-Parise is dated January 22, 1672. He died a little over two months later, March 30, 1672. Nothing is known of the nature of his last illness. He was buried on April 1, 1672, in the Church of St.-Germain l'Auxerrois, at eleven o'clock in the morning.

VOVS eſtes priez d'aßiſter au Convoy, Service & Enterrement de deffunt noble homme M^E Guy Patin, Conſeiller Medecin, Lecteur, & Profeſſeur du Roy au College Royal de France, & Docteur Regent en la Faculté de Medecine à Paris, decedé en ſa maiſon ruë du Chevalier du Guet; Qui ſe fera Vendredy premier iour d' Avril 1673 à vnze heures preciſes du matin, en l'Egliſe Saint Germain Lauxerrois ſa parroiſſe, où il ſera inhumés Les Dames s'y trouveront s'il leur plaiſt.

Vn De profundis.

INVITATION TO PATIN'S FUNERAL
(From Pierre Pic: Guy Patin, Paris, 1911)

BIBLIOGRAPHIC NOTES

The following is a list of the most important material bearing on Guy Patin, which has been used in the present study:

CABARET. Un docteur bibliophile condamné aux galéres perpétuelles. *Gaz. d. hop.* Par., 1855, xxviii, 93. [An interesting account of Charles Patin.]

CHEREAU, A. Quelques lettres inédites de Guy Patin. *Union Méd.*, Patin, 1876, 3rd ser., xxi, 949; xxii, 12; 49; 129; 165; 237; 309; 381; 453; 533; 621; 697. [Under the numbers 9357 and 9358 *du fonds français* in the department of manuscripts the Bibliothèque nationale possesses two portfolios of original letters of Guy Patin. These number 342, and were written between 1630 and 1670, 117 are addressed to the Belins of Troyes, 169 to Charles Spon of Lyons, and fifty-four to the Salins, father and son who practiced at Beauvais, one to Bachey, a physician of Beaume, and one to the son of Claude Saumaise. Besides these letters in the Bibliothèque nationale, Reveillé-Parise published 478 letters written by Patin to Falconet of Lyons. At the date when Chereau wrote (1876) it was not known where the originals were to be found. Chereau also states that from time to time unpublished letters of Guy Patin's are found in private collections or offered at public sales. They are regarded as rarities and bring high prices. Chereau publishes thirty-three letters in the course of these articles in the *Union Mêdicale*.]

CHEREAU, A. Bibliographie Patiniana—Catalogue chronologique, analytique et explicatif des ouvrages composés par Guy Patin, et de ceux à la publication desquels il a contribué. *Gaz. hebd. de méd. et dechir.*, Par., 1879, 2nd ser., xvi, 549; 565; 581. [After commenting on the curious fact that Patin's real literary output was so small compared with his intense interest in all literary matters, Chereau proceeds to list his writings as far as he had been able to identify them.

1. Cabinet des cantiques spirituels. Propres pour élever l'Âme à Dieu, recueillis des plusieurs Pères religieuses par G. P. B. Troisième part. A Paris, chez Anthoine de Sommaville, au Palais, en la galerie des Libraires, près la Chancellerie. 1623. Avec privilége du Roy. [One of the religious Canticles in this book is signed with Patin's initials and another with those of his father.]

2. Thèses written by Patin and disputed before the Faculté de Médecine de Paris.

A. First thèse quodlibétaire; December 19, 1624: *Estne feminae in virum mutatio αδυνατος?* Is the transformation of a woman into a man impossible? [Concluded in the affirmative.]

B. Second thèse quodlibétaire; November 27, 1625: *An praegnanti periculose laboranti abortus?* [Concluded in the affirmative.]

C. Thèse quodlibétaire proposed by George Joudounyn on December 16, 1627, but written by Patin and presided at by the latter. It was entitled: *Ergo μητρομανια balneum?* Are baths useful in uteromania? [Concluded in the affirmative.]

D. Patin presided again, December 17, 1643, at the thesis of the bachelor, Paul Courtois, for whom he not only chose the subject, but wrote the thesis entitled: *Estne totus homo à naturâ morbus?* Do all the diseases of man come from nature?

E. March 14, 1647, Guy Patin presided at the thèse cardinale of Jean de Montigny. To the thesis of Montigny, Patin added a disquisition of his own entitled: *Estne longae ac jucundae vitae tuta certaque parens sobrietas?* Is sobriety the most sure Mother of a long and agreeable life? [This was the thesis which got him into so much trouble with the apothecaries because of the fury with which he attacked them and their preparations. In it he said that antimony was *diabolicon inter remedia monstrum; vin émétique* was *venenato stibio infectum;* bezoar, *idolum fatuorum;* theriac, *compositio luxuriae;* mithridatum, *herbarum deforme chaos;* and confection of hyacinth and alkermes were *diamargaritum et Arabum pigmenta.* He said that these precious remedies were of no more use to cure diseases than lime or cinders, and that they were made by ignorant charlatans and birds of prey. The Apothecaries brought a process against him and it was in court on this occasion that he made his own defence with an eloquence which won him great applause and an acquittal.]

F. On December 8, 1670, Jean Cordelle read a thesis entitled: *Estne sanguis per omnes corporis venas et arterias jugiter circumfertur?* Is the blood carried without interruption by all the veins and arteries of the body? [Patin defended the negative side in a thesis which was published. Chereau quotes a sample of the opprobrious language used by Patin, and justly states that it affords a pathetic spectacle to find a man of Patin's professional standing attempting to deny a fact which had been so clearly proven forty-two years previously.]

G. In 1671 Patin presided at another thése cardinale of Jean Cordelle, and wrote for the occasion a thesis against the use of theriac as a remedy in pestilential fevers: *Estne theriaca pestilenti febre jactatis venenum?*

3. In 1628 there was published an edition of the works of Ambroise Paré on the title-page of which was the following statement: "Les oeuvres d'Ambroise Paré . . . Reveuës et corrigées en plusieurs endroits, et augmentée d'un fort ample Traicté des Fiebvres, tant en général, qu'en particulier, et de la curation d'icelles, nouvellement trouvé dans les manuscrits de l'autheur. Paris, Nicolas Buon, 1628." On November 4, 1631, Patin wrote to Belin: "The Paré of the last edition, wellbound, costs eight livres, without rebate. It is augmented in this last impression by a new treatise on fevers, which has been added at the end of the book, and is made by a physician *intus et in cute mihi noto*, without having put his name to it." [Chereau argues from the style of the treatise that the anonymous author was no other than Patin.]

4. In 1628 there was published at Paris an edition of the works of André du Laurens, translated into Latin from the French. The translator was Guy Patin and he also enriched the works of Henri IV's famous physician with numerous notes.

5. Enchiridion anatomique, compilé et dressé en bon ordre par M. Jean Vigier, corrigé et augmenté en cette dernière edition (par Guy Patin). Paris, J. Jost, 1630. [A small manual of anatomy.]

6. Traité de la conservation de la santé par un bon régime à légitime usage des choses requises pour bien et heureusement vivre. Paris, 1632. [This treatise on popular hygiene was published as an addendum to a work entitled "Le médecin charitable" by Philibert Guybert. It first appeared in the seventeenth edition of Guybert's book with a separate title page and pagination. The book was translated into Latin by G. Sauvagneon of Lyons and published with the title "Medicus officiosus."]

7. In 1635 an edition of the works of de Baillou was published at Paris, for which Patin compiled a copious analytical table of contents.

8. In 1637 Patin edited an edition of the "Orationes et Praefationes" of Jean Passerat, which was published at Paris.

9. In 1641 a syndicate of publishers of Paris published the works of Daniel Sennert. [Patin had not only stimulated them to the enterprise but edited the book and wrote the preface. Sennert had died four years previous to its publication.]

10. In 1614 Patin published a manuscript by P. Chanet, a physician of la Rochelle entitled "Considerations sur la sagesse de Charron." [The author had left the manuscript in Patin's charge.]

11. Several pamphlets on behalf of the Faculté de Médecine in its contest with Renaudot. [These were anonymous but Chereau identified them by the records of the Faculté, which show that Patin was deputed to write them.]

12. In 1648 Charles Guillemeau sustained a thesis, *Estne hippocratica medendi methodus omnium certissima, tutissima praestantissima?* Is not the Hippocratic method the most certain, surest, and most

excellent to cure the sick? [When Guillemeau published his thesis he asked Patin to add to it certain "Observations" and he did so, we may be sure, with delight.]

13. In 1648 he supervised the publication of the "Encheiridium anatomicum et pathologicum" of Riolan, and in 1653 his "Opera anatomica vetera recognita et auctiora." [As Chereau says these are the chief literary evidences of Patin's interest in anatomy, although in 1623 he was appointed *Archidiacre* of the schools of medicine in the University of Paris, a position equivalent to that of *chef des travaux anatomiques*, and in 1654 he was made Professor of anatomy and botany in the Collége de France.]

14. When Sauvagneon published the "Medicus officiosus," a Latin translation of the work of Philibert Guybert with Patin's "Traité de la conservation de la santé," he added to it a little treatise by Nicolas Ellain entitled "Avis sur la peste." At his request Patin wrote a number of notes on Ellain's work.

15. Sauvagneon also added to the "Medicus officiosus" a translation of a little treatise entitled, "Quelques notes sur un livre de Galien: 'De missione sanguinis,' livre traduit en français et commenté par Louis Savot." To this he also got Patin to add some notes and observations.

16. Gérard Denisot, who died in 1594, was not only a distinguished physician of the Faculté de Médecine but also a poet. At his death his library was purchased by an advocate named Joly. Among its contents he found the ms. of an elegant poetic version of the "Aphorisms" of Hippocrates in Greek and French verse, written by Denisot. This

ms. Joly presented to the Faculté de Médecine, accompanying the gift by a letter of presentation written in Greek. The gift was made during the *décanat* of Patin, in 1652. Patin translated Joly's letter into Latin and added to it some annotations about Denisot. The letter in Greek with Patin's translation was published in 1656 in a book entitled "Divers opuscules tirés des Memoires de M. Antoine Loysel . . . publies par Claude Joly . . . Par., 1656."

17. In the "Elogia" of Papyre Masson, published in 1656, those on Simon Pietre and François Miron were written by Patin.

18. Van der Linden of Leiden dedicated the edition of Celsus, which he published in 1657, to Patin, thanking him in the dedication for the great assistance he had lent him in the work. [Chereau does not state that Patin wrote any part of the book, but says that he lent Van der Linden all the various editions of Celsus which he possessed, many of them enriched by ms. notes by Fernel, and other savants.]

19. A Jesuit priest wrote a life of Galen, "Vita Claudii Galeni, Pergameni, medicorum principis, expropriis operibus collecta, per R. P. Phil. Labbeum . . . ad V. C. Guidonem Patinum . . . Paris 1660." [How Patin came to be willing to publish anything written by one of the Order he so heartily detested is not explained, but the fact remains that he did. Patin wrote Falconet (May 28, 1660): "The Father Phil. Labbé, a Jesuit, native of Bourges, has made a little volume of the life of our Galen, all taken from his works. He has given and dedicated it to me in ms. I am going to have it printed in octavo, and then we can send it to all our friends."]

20. Patin contributed many valuable notes and additions to the third edition of "La bibliographie médicale de Van der Linden," published at Amsterdam in 1662.

21. Patin was a great admirer of Gaspard Hoffmann. [When Hoffmann died, in 1648, he left an unpublished ms. which Patin purchased from his daughter for fifty *écus*. Although he got the ms. in 1649 Patin did not succeed in getting it published until eighteen years later, when it appeared with the title, "Apologia pro Galeno, sive *xpbΣto maθeiΩn* libri duo. ex bibliotheca Guidonis Patini."]

FOUCART. *Gaz. d. hop.* Par., 1847, 28., ix, 403. [A short account of his life with no originality.]

MONTANIER, H. *Gaz. d. hop.* Par., 1864, xxxvii, 93; 101; 113. [Gives an outline of his biography from the ordinary sources, and reviews many of his idiosyncrasies.]

PATIN, CHARLES. Lyceum Patavinum, sive icones et vitae professorum Patavii MDCL, xxxii, publice docentium. Pars trios, theologos, philosophos et medicos complectens. Patavii, 1682.

PIC, PIERRE. Guy Patin, avec 74 portraits ou documents, Paris, G. Steinheil, Éditeur, 1911.

Lettres choisies de feu Mr. Guy Patin, Docteur en médecine de la Faculté de Paris, & Professeur au Collége Royal. Dans lesquelles sont contenués plusieurs particularités historiques sur la vie & la mort des scavans de ce siècle, sur leurs écrits & plusieurs autres choses curieux depuis l'an 1645 jusque 1672. Augmentées de plus de 300 lettres dans cette derniére édition; et divisées en trois volumes; volume 1, A Cologne, chez Pierre du Laurens. MDCXCL.

Reveillé-Parise, J. H. Lettres de Guy Patin, nouvelle édition augmentée de lettres inédites, précédée d'un notice biographique, accompagnée de remarques scientifiques, historiques, philosophiques et littéraires, avec un portrait et le facsimile de l'écriture de Gui Patin, 3 vols. Paris, J. B. Ballière, 1846.

St. Ludgere, Moreau de. *Gaz. d. hop.* Par., 1839, 2nd ser., i, 293. [Brief *résumé* of Patin's life and opinions of no originality.]

Triaire, Paul. Lettres de Guy Patin, 1630–1672, nouvelle édition collationnée sur les manuscrits autographes, publiée avec l'addition des lettres inédites, la restauration des textes retranchés ou altérés, et des notes biographiques, bibliographiques, et historiques. Paris, Librairie Honoré Champion, 1907. [Only one volume has been published of this which promises to be the most complete and scholarly of all the editions of Patin's letters.]

INDEX OF PERSONAL NAMES